Praise for
The Seven Chakra Per[...]

"Life guidance as to 'why we are who we are.' Shai has made a great contribution to the vibrant living library of evolving human consciousness in a most integrated, readable, and admirable way. His insights encourage the reader to understand the deep connections between chakras, mind, body, and spirit. A must read."

—**Patricia Mercier,** author of bestselling
The Chakra Bible and *The Little Book
of Chakras*

"A magnificent way to understand yourself as a spiritual being having a physical experience. Highly recommended!"

—**C. Norman Shealy,** MD, PhD, author
of *Living Bliss: Major Discoveries Along
the Holistic Path*

"In an era in which we frequently limit our perspective of ourselves to a body, mind, or soul, this book is a wonderful invitation to experience yourself as an inspiring integration of all three."

—**Dr. Itai Ivtzan,** associate professor,
Naropa University, and mindfulness
teacher and researcher

"A new perspective of the chakras representing archetypal personalities. This integrative approach identifies and illuminates spiritual, mental, and emotional patterns that give clarity toward soul essence and personal path."

—**Francesca McCartney,** PhD,
Academy of Intuition Medicine

"A peaceful world starts with a peaceful mind, and this book encourages peace by helping us understand all facets of our being, helping us to embrace other points of view, and leading us to experience wholeness within ourselves."

—**Cindy Lora-Renard,** spiritual life coach
and author of *A Course in Health
and Well-Being*

the seven chakra
personality types

the seven chakra personality types

DISCOVER THE ENERGETIC FORCES
THAT SHAPE YOUR LIFE, YOUR RELATIONSHIPS,
AND YOUR PLACE IN THE WORLD

SHAI TUBALI

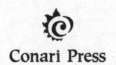

Conari Press

For permission requests, please contact the publisher at:
Mango Publishing Group
2850 S Douglas Road, 2nd Floor
Coral Gables, FL 33134 USA
info@mango.bz

For special orders, quantity sales, course adoptions and corporate sales, please email the publisher at sales@mango.bz. For trade and wholesale sales, please contact Ingram Publisher Services at customer. service@ingramcontent.com or +1.800.509.4887.

The Seven Chakra Personality Types: Discover the Energetic Forces that Shape Your Life, Your Relationships, and Your Place in the World

Library of Congress Cataloging-in-Publication Data is available on request.
ISBN: (print) 978-1-57324-736-8
BISAC category code: OCC010000, BODY, MIND & SPIRIT / Mindfulness & Meditation

Printed in the United States of America

Dedicated to my soul family:

Tamar, Noga, Alaya, Philipp, Mimi, Theresa, Jan, and Nir.

All of you are rays of the great sun, beautiful embodiments of your own chakra types.

CONTENTS

CONTENTS

ACKNOWLEDGMENTS

My heartfelt gratitude to Noga and Jan Müller, the managers of my Berlin center, who supported the writing process from beginning to end. They toiled tirelessly to build up the one-year school platform from which this book emerged.

I am profoundly thankful to Florian Stündel, who meticulously transcribed all the hundreds of hours of the school teachings, enabling me to refine them into the essential content of this book.

My deep gratitude also to my designer, Oliver Bruehl, for creating the two effective visual models found in these pages.

Finally, I humbly acknowledge the many participants of the 2017 Seven Chakra Types school. Your enthusiasm, intense questioning, and curiosity helped to deliver numerous insights that have greatly clarified this system.

PREFACE

The seven chakras (Sanskrit for "wheels" or "circles") belong to a Hindu system originating in India between 1500 and 500 BC, which makes it one of the oldest and most persistent systems the world has ever known. They were introduced by the seers of ancient India as seven major confluences within our subtle nerve network that also function as psychic centers of energy and consciousness. Each chakra relates to a set of energetic, emotional, mental, and spiritual activities. Thus each is a powerful determinant of all levels of human existence.

The chakras are often reduced to a simplistic set of seven energy centers known in the popular literature for their symbols and colors. This literature focuses, for the most part, on general principles of healing, balancing, and awakening. It generally presents only a superficial understanding of the chakras as centers of emotional energy and spiritual power.

At a deeper level, however, the chakras define seven centers of perception and experience. Through these centers, we each encounter and experience our own multidimensional reality. When you look at life through the lens provided by the chakras, you discover that life can be seen in specific and distinct ways, and in light of this discovery, different values, meanings, and happiness become far more relevant.

The chakra personality types derive from the seven different worldviews related to the seven individual chakras. Your own personality type depends on which center of perception—which chakra—is aroused most easily in you and most naturally gets in touch with reality before all others do. This intense identification with your chakra's perspective forms your most fundamental personality type—what I call your "major chakra type."

Within this broader context, the chakras show us how our so-called individual inclinations can be classified into seven types of perception and experience. Unfortunately, we are rarely introduced to the chakras as illuminators of our individual paths and as indicators of the way our individual journeys unfold or could unfold.

We all possess seven chakra energies that make up our human wholeness, although some are far more active and some are *relatively* negligible—not necessarily because we have neglected certain aspects of our being, but rather because we are inherently destined to embody and bring to full flowering one major aspect of life and the cosmos.

The system of personality types presented here is a development of fundamental principles found in yogic teachings. Throughout my years of theoretical and experiential research in the field of chakras, I began to notice suggestions of personality types that sprang from the individual chakras and that corresponded with unique perspectives. These suggestions—often brief and superficial—seemed to represent human archetypes that included animal symbolism—an ant representing the first chakra, a butterfly representing the second, and so on.

As I dug deeper into these correspondences, I came to realize that our individual differences and unique expressions all fall into seven major categories related to the seven chakras. Indeed, each category defined a world unto itself comprised of tendencies, attractions, and passions. A closer examination of this principle convinced me that each of us identifies with one major chakra and, to a lesser degree, with one or two other chakras.

This insight enabled me to appreciate the hidden elements behind all personalities—a sort of "soul design"—based on profound inclinations that, when fulfilled, make each of us feel happier and more complete than in any other possible condition in life. This is the system I present to you here.

CHAKRA PERSONALITY TYPE IN WORLD POPULATION

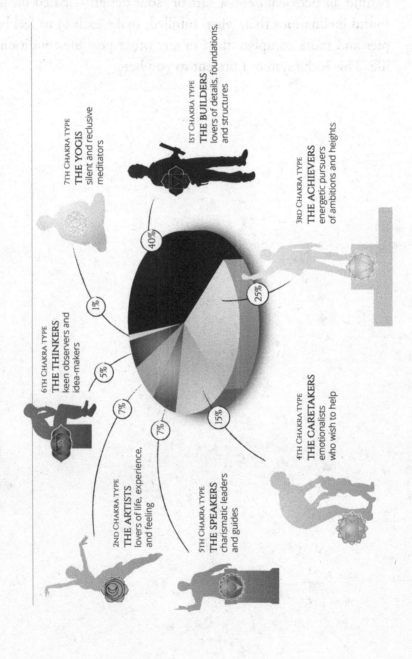

7TH CHAKRA TYPE
THE YOGIS
silent and reclusive
meditators

1ST CHAKRA TYPE
THE BUILDERS
lovers of details, foundations,
and structures

3RD CHAKRA TYPE
THE ACHIEVERS
energetic pursuers
of ambitions and heights

6TH CHAKRA TYPE
THE THINKERS
keen observers and
idea-makers

2ND CHAKRA TYPE
THE ARTISTS
lovers of life, experience,
and feeling

5TH CHAKRA TYPE
THE SPEAKERS
charismatic leaders
and guides

4TH CHAKRA TYPE
THE CARETAKERS
emotionalists
who wish to help

40%
1%
25%
5%
7%
7%
15%

INTRODUCTION
CHAKRAS AND PERSONALITY

What makes you feel the happiest and most complete in life? Surely, you can come up with more than one thing, but try to get in touch with the most fulfilled moments you have ever had. Was it an unimaginable depth of intimacy and love you shared with a soul mate? Or was it a moment in which you felt that you managed to crack open the secrets of the universe? Was it a silent retreat in some far-off spot in the Himalayas? Or perhaps an electrifying speech you gave to a responsive audience, a truly adventurous journey around the world, a tremendous leap you made in your career, or designing and building your own dream house?

Whatever has made you feel most happy and fulfilled in life is most likely a function of your chakra type. What does that mean? Your chakra type determines the way you perceive and experience the world. It leads you to pay attention to particular elements in your life while hardly noticing others. It draws you to those elements in your life that you intuitively feel are the most meaningful and most essential for your happiness.

More often than not, we simply explain our individual differences by pointing out that we all have our own inclinations. Different strokes for different folks. On the other hand, there are many systems for self-knowledge in the world that have attempted to crack open the mystery of our individuality and determine why each of us experiences life so differently. These systems strive to help us understand why we each have certain inclinations and tendencies, why we suffer from certain excesses and deficiencies, certain frustrations and anxieties, and how we apply our individual skills and abilities. Some, like psychoanalysis, are based entirely on individual history, tracing our anxieties back to traumatic incidents that occurred at the age of three. Others—like numerology, enneagrams, and human-design techniques—classify human tendencies and behavior into general and universal categories. The system of chakra types, the ancient system that offers us a profound and illuminating answer of its own, belongs to this latter group.

Chakras and the Individual

No question, everyone is destined to fully realize all seven chakras in order to embody a fully balanced and fully realized human being. None of us can turn our backs on the challenges and trials in life that fulfill each chakra's psychological role, nor should we avoid the development of all qualities and powers inherent in each of the seven. But it is impossible for any of us, even the most advanced beings imaginable, to manifest all of life's aspects. Though this may sound limiting, it is actually quite beautiful. This is why we have different expressions of the same experience.

It is clear that we all have a unique perspective on life. For this reason, even when we share the same experiences, we tend to interpret and express them very differently. Perhaps the most striking demonstration of this is found in the intensely different expressions of the state of spiritual enlightenment, which is said to be singular and yet the same for all.

Rumi, the great Sufi poet and mystic, spoke of love of the divine, and of surrender and union. Gurdjieff, the Armenian master, focused on willpower, on overcoming, and on self-remembrance. Osho, Jiddu Krishnamurti, and Ramana Maharshi had clearly distinct approaches that led to very different paths and practices. These differences of interpretation and expression derived from the different chakra personality types to which each belonged. This chakra type acted as a prism that caused the divine light that shone through them to be expressed as a distinct ray of light rather than as the full spectrum of divine illumination. This "fragmentation" enables myriad individual experiences of the same "life" to come into being.

Your personality type defines your most essential and persistent worldview. It has nothing to do with specific phases of your life in which you need to focus more on developing certain abilities and qualities or on answering important challenges. At times, you may find yourself needing to open your heart more, or to cultivate your independence, or strengthen your ground. Indeed, realizing that some part of you is more important than others at a certain stage of your life is an inevitable part of your whole-human development and balance.

In the same way, your personality type may not be related to certain strengths you naturally possess. You can be generous, willful, or meditative without it being an indication of your type. Locating your personality means recognizing your basic constitution—the fundamental way in which you perceive and experience life, and your most fundamental attractions and passions. It is about the way you meet reality and the way you use it to harness the forces of your constitution and fulfill your destiny. Another way to think of it is as the impulse or inclination that you find irresistible because it stems from your most authentic self. This impulse may have such a strong pull that, at times, it feels bigger than yourself. When followed, it can easily engage you in a way that makes you nearly forget everything else.

Your chakra type does not necessarily correspond with what you do in your life at the moment or what you want to think of yourself. It is not even found in tendencies you deem admirable. Personally, I admire Mother Teresa—but that doesn't mean I am a fourth-chakra type. It may actually imply that she reflects to me certain aspects that are harder for me to fulfill. That is why the best method is to follow the way you first meet with the world. What is the first center in you that responds to things you encounter? Is it the mental part, your cognition and understanding? Or is it feeling, emotion, or will?

A helpful key is the fact that the seven personality types are divided into three major groups of perception and experience: the material-earthly types, the emotional-communicative types, and the mental-spiritual types. The first, second, and third chakras belong to the first group; the fourth and fifth chakras belong to the second; and the sixth and seventh chakras belong to the third. These groupings are based on how each type most directly experiences the world and what it initially arouses in them. The first or so-called "lowest" group—"lowest" only in terms of its location on the body, not its place in a hierarchy—initially meets the world through the senses and perceivable objects. The second group first encounters the world through emotions and fantasies. The third does not really directly experience the world at all. They meet it more as an idea and translate experience into abstract principles.

Your Chakra Type

The journey offered in this book is a colorful and vivid one. This is because it doesn't deal merely with big abstract principles of spirituality, but rather with very particular, richly nuanced, partly funny individual realities—the realities of human nature as reflected in the chakra system. The more you read through the book, the more you will notice that you spontaneously identify with the ways you think and behave according to the types—and with the ways your friends, partners, and children think and behave. You will realize that we all fall into one of the seven major patterns as different perceivers and experiencers of reality. Recognizing these seven patterns is the beginning of learning how to control and optimize them more effectively.

At a certain point, you will also begin to classify other experiences into these seven patterns—for instance, while watching a movie, or looking at a certain advertisement, or participating in a lecture. Since our culture—religion, art, entertainment—consists entirely of the contributions of the seven types, it is only natural that all cultural phenomena will bear the distinct orientation and focus of one of them. The system of chakra types thus provides a healthy way to understand and appreciate our human diversity, as well as a way to promote self-knowledge, tolerance, and openness. Through its lessons, we become better receivers of the gifts each chakra type has to offer.

More often than not, people think that their perception of the world is the same as everyone else's. That is why we always seem so surprised when someone completely disagrees with our own worldview. But the system of chakra personality types reveals to us that everyone does *not* see the same world. Sometimes, we need to embrace the worldview of others to enhance our own experience and to supply aspects that may be missing from our own perception. This is important to understand, because my vision of the seven types is not hierarchical in any way; rather, it is communal. When I describe each type in detail, my clear aim is not only to help you recognize your own special self, but also to make you appreciate all seven types. I wish everyone to see the world through the eyes of each chakra type and to appreciate this vision as an essential ingredient of their own being.

The most direct way to locate your own chakra type is to read through the chapters that outline each of the types carefully and try to recognize whether you have just read a description of yourself. Sooner or later, you will encounter a profile so intimate and comfortably familiar that something in you will leap forward and declare, "Hey, he is talking about me!" This chakra is most likely your major personality type.

Finding your major personality type shouldn't feel like guessing. You may find yourself a little torn between two types—in fact, this may actually be an important indication of something we will discuss later—but eventually one will gain the upper hand and make you feel that you are coming home, as if you recognize your very own way of seeing the world. This, by the way, can be a somewhat amusing and self-revealing process, during which you will feel embarrassingly transparent.

Other chapters—perhaps one or two—will seem to describe "close relatives" of your personality, containing reasonably large parts of your being, yet still not feeling like a perfect fit. These chakras are most likely your secondary and supportive personality types. Most chapters, however, will seem totally foreign to you, or perhaps may seem to be a better fit for your partner or for someone you know.

That said, it is important to clarify what you should be looking for in this process. The description closest to yourself needs to feel intimate and familiar, not merely because you have recognized certain behavioral patterns or positive and negative attributes, as you might find some part of your personality in an astrological or numerological chart. Remember, this system is about recognizing your heart's deepest calling, so you must look for the constitution that most easily fits you and in which you can best fulfill your own soul design.

That is why, even in the description of your major chakra type, you are not expected to embrace every little detail. What determines your chakra type is the lens through which you perceive the world. This lens makes you notice certain elements while overlooking others, and thus determines what is most meaningful and valuable to you. The question you must ask yourself as you read through these chapters is, "Is this the way I experience life?"

Some small details can be eliminated from your personality for the simple fact that none of us is purely and perfectly one major chakra type. Types that feel like your personality's close relatives also have a role in shaping your life. Don't be concerned, for instance, if you recognize yourself when you read that another type finds it hard to wake up in the morning and start a new day.

You also shouldn't expect that your major chakra type will contain all of your strengths and talents. Just because you belong to one chakra type doesn't mean that you cannot come into the world equipped with various qualities and capacities from different chakras, or that you won't develop these qualities along the way. Your type is all about what you *love* the most—that which gives the most intimate experience of yourself.

Of course, sometimes your true chakra type may be buried beneath thick layers of suppression, social adaptations, or certain life conditions. This makes the process of self-discovery a deep probing of your most fundamental soul elements that gradually encourages your chakra type to rise from beneath the thick layers of concealment and declare itself. In the same way, you can become trapped in a severely unbalanced expression of your type that demonstrates its more constrained forms.

Moreover, superficial guessing can lead you astray, because you may already expect or want to be a certain type because it better suits your self-image or some cherished lifestyle habits. If you fear this is the case for you, you may need more than your own direct reading to give you perspective. One way to get this perspective is by answering questions like the ones you will find at the end of each chapter. These questions can help you by pinpointing key qualities and behaviors that are more crucial than others in determining the type. If you are still uncertain, you may want to have a private session with an expert in the field who can give you a qualified outsider's analysis. In my own private sessions, I use a technique called "chakra reflection" that reveals which of a person's chakras contains the highest energy concentration—a subtler expression of mental and emotional identification with chakra type.

Children's Chakra Types

Finding the chakra type of children can sometimes be a challenge. Some children show defined chakra characteristics at early stages in life. If you have a child so strongly defined, it is quite easy to guess his or her type. However, in most cases, it is difficult to be certain, for the simple reason that it is during childhood that the fragile and fragmented personality begins to consolidate. During childhood and adolescence, some of the chakra centers are in a state of rapid development, which makes observing children's and teenagers' tendencies quite confusing. The general development of the chakras can get mixed up with the expression of a child's unique chakra type. You have to penetrate the veils of psychological maturation to find a persistent line of tendencies and attractions.

Moreover, while some children and teenagers are more defined than others and stand out in skills and tendencies, the majority of them are in an intense process of self-searching and self-definition and may only contact their dormant talents and passions in later stages of life. For most people, it takes a lot of time and many life experiences to attain a stable unfolding of their chakra type.

Thus, while guessing is always fun, determining chakra type with complete certainty is safest when the person is between the ages of twenty-one and twenty-eight. These ages are not arbitrary. In chakra development, each period of seven years constitutes a cycle of life during which a certain chakra matures. Thus, by the age of twenty-one, a person has attained a basic foundation of the three lower chakras, which means their basic personality is more or less established.

Your Three-Type Structure

If you find yourself torn between two chakra types, don't be concerned. This just means that you have encountered both your major personality type and a secondary type. Now you must determine which is dominant. Which one is your true self?

The good news is that there is a simple self-test you can use to help you do that. You will find one at the end of each chapter. Just follow the instructions to estimate the percentage of the specific chakra type in you. This percentage is not estimated in relation to other types. You simply evaluate the degree of presence of a chakra type in your personality on a scale of 1 to 100. In other words, how much of all that you read about the chakra type feels close to your being. After reading through all seven chapters and evaluating each type in this way, gather all the percentages and determine which chakra type received the highest score. The one with the highest score is your major personality type. You may find that one of the seven chakra types is so strikingly identical to your own experience that you give it a perfect score of 100 percent. But even a score of "only" 90 or 80 percent may indicate your major type, as long as it is your highest score.

Even if you recognize yourself as belonging 100 percent to a certain type, however, in reality no one is truly 100 percent of any type. For instance, in Ayurvedic medicine, an ancient Hindu system built around the central concept of three fundamental elements or energies called *doshas* that circulate in the body and govern all physiological activity, it is the balance between these elements that determines health and disease. *Vata* (air) controls all movement; *pitta* (fire) regulates heat and intensity; *kapha* (water) is responsible for nourishment. Each individual possesses different proportions of these elements, which are the cause of individual physical constitution and temperament, including particular dispositions to certain physical and mental tendencies and disorders. But no person is 100 percent pitta or 100 percent vata or 100 percent kapha. Each individual consists of an endlessly varied combination of these elements.

In the same way, although each individual has a major chakra personality type, all of humanity is obviously not strictly divided into seven types. The seven major chakra types are too archetypal to include all the subtleties and nuances of an actual living personality. That is why each complete personality is made up of a major type, as well as a second type and a supportive type. These secondary and supportive personality types endow us with more distinct characteristics and make our personalities unique. They add a perspective and life experience that completes your major type. Your second highest score on the self-test indicates your secondary chakra type; your third highest score indicates your supportive chakra type. Together, these three chakra types form a sort of trinity whose interaction captures very successfully your life's journey and purpose.

Your second and supportive personality types, when combined with your major type, help to define you as a complete individual—one who is balanced, rounded, and empowered by the interaction between the three types. This is the beauty and wisdom of the chakra-type system. It allows for the description of many diverse individual personalities through the creative combination of chakra characteristics. These combinations may be a source of inner conflict and tension for those they describe, but they also give rise to unique personalities.

By combining the seven major types in a threefold structure, the chakra personality system provides for an elaborate mapping of forty-two distinct personality types. And since each personality consists of interaction between three dominant chakra types, an amazing 252 personality types can be mapped. Factor into this the relative proportion of the percentages of each of the three chakras, and you have an almost limitless array of personality types to consider.

Fulfilling Your Chakra Type

Knowing your three-type personality structure does more than add one more factor to your self-image or vaguely support your feelings and intuitions about yourself. When you learn about your constitution, you can harness its powers and direct it toward an ideal fulfillment of your soul design. That is why, at the end of each of the following chapters, you will find suggestions for lifestyle changes that deal with everything from very small and mundane details, to broader emotional, mental, and behavioral issues, to profound spiritual enlightenment. By following these suggestions, you can tune into a fully realized model of your type. You do this by balancing the excesses of your type and encouraging its natural fulfillment.

As a rule, each chakra type wants to do precisely those things that lead to imbalance. And the great irony is that, usually, what seems healthy to a chakra type is precisely what is the most unbalanced. Indeed, balancing your chakra energies may seem a bit like taming your personality type rather than letting it freely spread its wings. But unless you tame your type, it can never properly and safely mature.

Each type has its own unbalancing elements that, when wrongly channeled, can lead to self-destruction and even psychosomatic disorders. That is why learning to harness your tendencies is vital to fulfilling your chakra type. Think of this balancing process as finding ways to express your nature within clear structures. These structures no doubt limit the flow of your expression, but they are, paradoxically, exactly what allows it to stream healthily out of your being—like directing a gushing river into channels that keep the flow active and, at the same time, manageable.

Eating a delicious food is wonderful in reasonable quantities. If you eat a whole cake, however, you may end up with a stomachache. To enjoy an experience, you must limit it. It is a part of the wisdom of life that unlimited or unregulated experience cannot be held or contained. Even your natural energy should best flow only at certain times and for certain uses. It should also ideally be directed less toward immediate forms of fulfillment and more toward genuinely constructive and lasting ends.

Imagine your chakra type as a wild horse that you don't yet know how to ride. It is not behaving badly; it is just improperly guided. You must find the right way to convince the horse to follow directions. The sections in each chapter on balance answer the following question in different ways and on different levels: What are the healthiest channels I can find to release the excesses of my tendencies and balance them?

Fulfilling the dormant potential of your chakra type is another challenge. In the sections in each chapter on fulfillment, you will find a set of suggestions that are meant to promote in you a genuine self-love—the kind that makes it possible for you to make peace with yourself, accept your constitution, and faithfully develop it despite social pressures to adapt to a more general pattern. These recommendations include individually tailored practices, daily structures and activities, and even spiritual paths that can lead to an acknowledgment of your true inclinations. Think of these sections as a map you can follow to find the most creative and fulfilling ways to express your personality and attain its higher destiny. Following these guidelines can help you transform your own strengths and talents into gifts you can share with the world.

At the core of the psychological structure, each personality type confronts certain challenges that create struggles within themselves and with reality—a kind of constant quarrel or resistance that needs to be recognized consciously and sorted out. Carl Jung called these aspects the "shadow self." I give each of these shadow selves a name and include them in the personality profiles that are covered in each chapter. The first chakra struggles with what I call the "frozen self," while the second risks becoming "the butterfly that gives nothing." The third type can be trapped as a "failure-fearing doer," while the fourth struggles with their tendency to be "rejected givers." Fifth-chakra types are threatened by their tendency to be "all-controlling manipulators," while sixth-chakra types can devolve into "helpless intellectuals." Seventh-chakra types have a propensity to withdraw that can lead them to become "anti-life meditators." Since these struggles and challenges are more easily noticed than our more subtle tendencies and attractions, which are sometimes heavily suppressed, recognizing them can be a powerful way to identify, with certainty, your major personality type.

In addition to these shadow selves, each personality type has weaknesses—certain aspects in which they are far less capable because those capacities are missing from the natural constitution of their personalities. To compensate for these weaknesses, we often make them into a matter of pride, as if they represented some great quality rather than a weakness. When we do this, we make our personality type a form of escape from uncomfortable and important challenges in our lives. These weaknesses are discussed with relation to each type in the chapters that follow.

Another component of your personality type relates to the specific emotional shocks and disappointments that each type tends to register more than others. Indeed, each personality type is affected by certain negative tendencies and experiences that other types may not even notice. This is why some memories leave deeply engraved imprints on us, while we dismiss other negative experiences as merely passing inconveniences.

These three components—your shadow self, your weaknesses, and your emotional shocks—lead you to certain psychological attitudes and inclinations that help to define who you are. But the good news is that none of these psychological structures have to remain as they are. Through sincere inner work, you can transform your personality structure in positive ways. That said, don't be too impatient with your structure. Remember, your main challenges provide the friction that helps you develop a more satisfying life. By constantly attempting to overcome them, you change along the way.

While the primary goal of this book is to help you discover your own chakra identity, I also recommend that you use the system you find here to explore that which may seem foreign to you. For this reason, in each chapter, I have included some thoughts on the role each type plays in the world and why society needs each type. Once you come to realize the gifts of each type, it becomes easier to recognize how each one can inspire you and enrich your own life. We must not forget that, in the end, as complete human beings, all of us are meant to have all the chakra types awakened in us. Learning from those who have capacities different from your own can help you see the world from a different perspective.

Practice waking up in the morning as a different type. Acting out this type's perspective and experience for one day from within its personality can be highly illuminating. We tend to forget that we don't have to be ourselves all the time. Truth be told, when we are only ourselves, we begin to lose touch with certain perspectives and responses to life that could solve some of our most nagging problems. What might happen in your life if you let a worldview of another type penetrate your vision? What if you were able to insert this personality into your being momentarily? Would it positively alter your usual way of coping with challenges? Can you find a certain gift that you need from another type's reservoir of skills and capacities? Could any of them awaken some dormant and much-needed part in you?

I present each group of chakras separately to give a deeper appreciation of the tendencies and attitudes specific to each one. Within each chapter, I have provided a profile of the chakra type that includes its strengths and potential, as well as its shadow self and its sphere of influence. Use these profiles to become aware of ways in which you can change and begin to realize your full potential. Each chapter also discusses the essence, constitution, history, worldview, and characteristics of the personality type to which it corresponds, along with suggestions for balancing and fulfilling each type. The self-test at the end of each chapter will help you evaluate your own chakra type. In Part IV, you'll find ways to use this knowledge to affect your lifestyle, your relationships, and your place in the world. I hope these tools will help you recognize and fulfill your own personality in ways that will enrich your experience and that of others.

PART I

Material-Earthly Types

The first, second, and third chakras all fall into the category of the material-earthly types. This group is the one most dedicated to working with the materials and objects of sensory perception. However, while they are all deeply engaged in the world of matter, each of these three chakra types approaches it from an extraordinarily different angle. This group corresponds with the lower part of the human form: the legs, the base of the spine, and the genitals and belly.

CHAPTER I

FIRST CHAKRA

The Builders

The Builders

» **Presence in world population:** around 40 percent

» **Public domain:** legal institutions, police, banks, cities, bureaucracy, health institutions, construction work, insurance companies

» **Typically found among:** policemen, lawmakers, accountants, doctors, programmers, technicians, construction workers, cartographers, secretaries

» **Dosha constitution:** kapha (water)

» **Dominated by:** the instinctual center, survival instinct, the physical body

» **Shadow self:** the frozen self

» **Time zone:** cyclical time

» **Traditional animal:** ant, elephant

» **Famous figures:** the biblical Moses, Confucius, Hammurabi, Hippocrates, Phidias, Muhammad al-Idrisi, Amerigo Vespucci, Maimonides, Mimar Sinan, Samuel Johnson, Samuel Hahnemann, Fibonacci, Immanuel Kant, Emmy Noether, Kort Godel, Alan Turing, Charles Darwin, Jonas Salk, Katherine Johnson, Frank Lloyd Wright

We start our journey into the seven personality types with the first chakra, whose type tends to be far more serious than the second type and far less ambitious than the third. Just like the foundational physical chakra they embody, first-chakra personalities constitute the solid base of world population. These people are Builders—lovers of detail and structure—and they are in charge of the material and earthly plane. Four out of every ten people are first-chakra types, and their impressive number reflects their fundamental role in human society. They tend to be the most "earthly" of the first group—the ones closest to the ground. However, this also means that—for better or worse—they are the closest to the laws of matter.

Essence

The first chakra is located in the perineum. Its region of influence extends to the legs and the base of the spine. It holds within it the essence of cosmic order and structure. Structure is the very foundation of life. Without it, no life could ever be manifested and expressed. The most immediate example of this is the structure of the human form—subatomic particles form atoms; atoms form molecules; molecules form cells; cells form organs; and organs form the physical body that allows you to read this book. All of these structural components are the building blocks that contain and sustain the life that is you.

On a far larger scale, the divine reality is, first of all, expressed as the cosmos's astounding order. Within infinite space, there are countless structures—galaxies, suns, planets, plants, and animals—that function as containers of the various forces and energies of life. We all know that, to hold water, we need a glass; in a similar way, to hold life, we need structures. To this end, the all-organizing hidden reality created forms and defined structures that could conduct energy and contain life. And for each system of matter and life, there is also a suitable set of laws that govern and operate it. Our bodies obey these laws, just as cosmic constellations obey their own laws. These laws, like those of gravity and relativity, keep everything in harmony.

Try, for a moment, to connect to the sense that everything in the universe is comprised of and contained by structures, forms, and laws. Even this book required careful structuring and a logical framework. If I had written spontaneously, without restraining my creative impulse or containing my inspiration within a structure, it would most likely fail to convey my ideas properly.

To build anything constructive in life, you must define a certain structure composed of a clear schedule, careful details, and small daily actions. Within this structure, you establish the flow of your days, weeks, months, and even years. In your home, you create a physical structure of floor and ceiling, walls, doors, and windows, in order to feel protected and to provide an environment in which you can live and express yourself. In fact, all of your material life is contained within structures.

Complementing the structures that hold all material life is matter itself: substance, density, volume, and weight. Visible matter is mostly solid, not airy. It is, obviously, *material* enough to achieve substance. That is why yogis of the past associated the first chakra with the heavy and robust being of the elephant. Other beings on earth that reflect this essence are whales and massive, ancient trees like sequoias and redwoods.

The first-chakra essence is also seen in the colonizing instincts of some organisms—for instance, ants, termites, and bees. These insects naturally form colonies composed of many physically connected, interdependent individuals. They combine their forces to work as one entity, busily and diligently dedicating all their energies to the greater good. Likewise, our bodies function as communities of atoms, molecules, and cells, with every particle contributing to the greater whole.

These three components—order and structure, dense matter, and colonizing instincts—are all essential characteristics of a first-chakra type. Now try to imagine a human being rising out of this essence.

Constitution

Builders are proud representatives of the kapha (water) element of the dosha system. Indeed, for better or worse, they are its human manifestation. Kapha energy is heavy, solid, steady, slow, and sometimes even static. It is the element that bears the materials of the body and is responsible not only for the physical structure of the body—tissues, muscles, bones, marrow, and joints—but also for substances like the internal organs, blood, and fat.

Think of Builders as the kapha element in human form. This type has quite an earthly appearance. They are generally grounded and heavy, with a solid constitution that tends to overweight. Their eyes are soft, and they are generally quiet and gentle people. They are also relatively slow, in movement and slow to react. This doesn't mean that they are inefficient, however. They just need to take their time in responding to people and events.

As we know from the need for balance, each essence can also appear in excess in each type. In the case of first-chakra types, this tendency is even worse, because they are purely kapha without a balancing element. Thus, they may easily become overly grounded, tired, and even lethargic.

Sphere of Influence

Since this personality type originates in the world of cosmic order and law, they are most often found pursuing roles in legal institutions where laws are formed and enforced. With billions of people moving around in one shared space, regulation is needed to prevent general chaos. And this is where first-chakra types exert their influence. They work to clarify limits of movement, behavior, and action, and help to define each individual's expected contribution to the greater whole. They give shape to right relationships between people and between social and political entities. They restrain competing forces and ensure that everyone has a place in the public domain. Indeed, we owe the entire structure of society and culture to first-chakra types—the Builders.

Builders constitute 40 percent of the world population. Though this is most certainly not an accurate statistical evaluation, it is fair to estimate that, among every ten people, four will be Builders. We should all be happy about that, because they hold the structures of the world together. We must never take these diligent creators of order for granted.

We do tend to undervalue them, however. It is a great irony that the most fundamental chakra type is also the one we appreciate least. This is because they are the least "romantic," poetic, or colorful type. They are the caretakers of all the small details that may seem boring and gray. But without them, the entire material world would collapse. Like children who fail to appreciate their parents' hardships and efforts to provide for all their enjoyment and peace of mind, we tend to overlook the work of the Builders in structuring our world.

Builders don't feel at all that what they do is boring, however. From their perspective, it appears quite fascinating. Indeed, a first-chakra type, in response to the accusation that their work is boring, would probably answer that that is not the worst trait someone could have. In their minds, there are far worse tendencies—like drifting through life and being so ungrounded that your entire well-being could, all of a sudden, become severely endangered.

Everything we see around us and take for granted—our well-built houses and carefully tended gardens, the dishes and cutlery in our kitchens, the food that awaits us in abundance in the supermarkets, our well-crafted furniture, our carefully paved roads, the infrastructure of our cities, our hospitals and cathedrals, our financial system, and so much more—is the handiwork of silent, sometimes almost invisible Builders. We notice and appreciate artists, charismatic politicians, and ambitious billionaires. But the platforms on which they give their speeches or display their creations, and the active systems that manage their affairs, are all the work of Builders.

The unusual insight that first-chakra types have into tools and machines of all kinds—from computers to cars—draws them to anything technical. This type is also found among those who gather data, like accountants, bankers, statisticians, cartographers, librarians, and secretaries. They take great joy in working with numbers and in sorting out streams of information, collecting all the elements that constitute the foundation of daily life. As lovers of all things earthly, they are also commonly found among farmers and those who work the land. They are particularly in tune with the land's predictable rhythms and cycles, and are happy to take care of something so reassuringly repetitive.

Builders often partake in some form of lawmaking and so are present in all types of legal institutions. They may also be attracted to forms of law enforcement and often work as lawyers—not necessarily in showy courtroom proceedings, but rather in quiet, steady work that deals with the finest details and nuances of the law. They also work in the medical world as doctors and researchers who are fascinated with the many intricate laws of human anatomy and physiology. Since they love testing substances and their effects, they are drawn to study different types of medicines, pharmaceuticals, supplements, and foods to determine how the body reacts to them. Thus they often work as nutritionists and alternative-medicine therapists. Simply put, wherever Builders recognize an order they can follow or contribute to, they will be there.

Builders don't like being eccentric or standing outside accepted structures. They are conformists, and usually place themselves in conventional frameworks of belonging and service. They feel much healthier when they affiliate themselves with established systems, because these systems have grown out of a long tradition of proven and tested wisdom. They are keen on supporting and perfecting the well-established foundations of society. That is why they often take a role in churches, parliaments, courtrooms, and banks. Their traditional bent attracts them to ancient lineages, so they often appear within religious traditions, where they are the ones who strive to preserve the original law.

Role in Human History

In a way, first-chakra types were the first humans on earth. Their first role was to inspect nature's elements, assess the threats of predators and natural disasters, and determine the best ways to tame a hostile environment. They were the ones who tried out different materials, foods, and housing options, searching for the most useful elements and the most livable environments. Indeed, our current pampered lifestyle is the result of countless first-chakra types who toiled tirelessly to improve the systems of human life.

Builders paved the way to the brave new worlds that more inspired and daring types pushed to reveal. While they were not courageous visionaries who were willing to take risks and to live unsettling and insecure lives, they were most certainly the ones who confronted the new reality and quickly began to put everything in order: "Here we will put this and there we will put that." After organizing everything, they formulated laws to preserve their structures and regulate living to the smallest detail imaginable.

Builders were the "elders" who came up with the concept of a lawful society. In any religious tradition, they were the ones who helped formulate the rules. In Judaism, for example, they were surely responsible for writing large parts of the Old Testament, with its tradition of commandments and laws—a catalog of dos and don'ts full of countless minor details. In later scriptures, these commandments were passionately discussed, commented on, and even expanded.

Worldview

First-chakra types see the world as a space in which to build. To them, there is no greater meaning in life than the one found in steady and persistent construction, improving the foundations and strengthening the roots of human society and culture. The material world and all its substances are here to be organized, arranged, and reshaped to form a harmonious and life-supporting environment.

Builders are not interested in the abstract and, for the most part, are not intensely philosophical or insightful. They are lovers of the material and objective world, attracted to forms and shapes and anything that can become tangible and straightforward realities. They are fascinated by the deep intelligence of matter and the beauty of material patterns. As they survey their surroundings, they immediately spot any elements that can make its infrastructure even better. They are always drawn to ways to make everything more workable and livable.

In many respects, the passion of the Builders to improve their environment is similar to the perseverance and persistence of billions of years of evolution, which works with a great yet steady force to improve physical forms. To build a fully functioning world requires this kind of persistence—a steady gathering of the unorganized mass of creation to bring it into an organized state. Thus we can think of first-chakra types as organizers who want to put everything in order. As organizers, they cannot stand discontinuity. In fact, they perceive chaos merely as a potential for a better order.

Builders see everything as useful. Any material is an opportunity to bring more order out of chaos. That is why they can be deeply fascinated by technicalities. They are enthralled by the workings of machines. As children, they perhaps tried to dismantle TVs and clocks to understand their inner workings and to challenge themselves with the task of putting them back together again.

First-chakra types are not really interested in the "why" of things. To them, this kind of thinking is an impractical contemplation that leads to no clear resolutions. Their enthusiasm, even if they are religious or spiritual, turns far less to questions of "why" than it does to questions of "how." They don't ask why the world was created, because they are far more interested in how the world works. What are its fundamental laws? And how can we improve them?

Since this is a world of action, to get something done we cannot rely on the brightness of vision or the excitement of a sudden impulse. What we truly require is the establishment of constant patterns of behavior and action based on the qualities of steadiness, perseverance, and diligence. When we have our heads in the clouds, we accomplish nothing. In the material world, only a slow, persistent effort can affect reality. We need to wake up in the morning knowing exactly what we are meant to do and obediently follow a list of duties until, at a certain point, results begin to appear.

Guided by the wish to see the world around them in order—and, to them, an orderly world is a beautiful world—Builders move forward steadily, step by step, taking into consideration the smallest details imaginable. After all, their entire worldview is made of these details; if any of them are overlooked, the whole structure might collapse. Think of accountants who go carefully through endless numbers, or contractors who know that a slight error in construction could cost lives. This kind of responsibility requires great care and constant checking and rechecking, because only this slow persistence allows for precision.

Builders are drawn to long-term projects that demand taking a deep, deep breath. They trust this type of persistent action in the world and are very suspicious of anything that seems too fiery and thrilling. They firmly believe that only goals and aims that require stamina are worthwhile and count in the end.

First-chakra personalities live with a sense of time as continuity—past, present, and future. They experience time as cyclical. To them, everything is measured by cycles: the passage of weeks or years, rites of passage, and repetitive celebrations and holy days. It feels so right to them that these occasions repeat themselves and that everyone gathers around for them. These rituals encourage a feeling that there is always something to which they can return.

Builders often envision the world as an inherent divine order to which we must conform in our actions and our way of life. Human society must be woven around this inherent order through the creation of a lawful and honorable spirit among people. A society's purpose is to merge itself into this order and to strive to manifest it. "As above, so below." When Builders behold the innate order, they feel obliged to make the earth as orderly and well-balanced as the heavens. God is, to them, the perfect cosmic order, sometimes even taking the form of a guiding father figure to whom they owe faithful obedience.

For first-chakra personalities, meaning and happiness lie in achieving consistent security and stability. They want to find a place where they belong; they want to belong to a family or tribe. This is particularly crucial to their psychological health. Other types may also develop strong attachments to family, but to Builders, family *is* happiness. The family unit represents completion and wholeness, and it is an essential component of their well-being. That is why they often don't consider family and home as just a space to return to at the end of the day. For them, it is the very purpose of life. This is where the experience of love awaits them. When they suffer the loss of a dear one, they are devastated and only take comfort in believing that they will be reunited in an afterlife.

In the Western world, first-chakra types mourn for the loss of communal life. For them, the individualistic, isolated life is not intuitive at all. They long for an actual sense of community. In its absence, they compensate by identifying themselves with their nations, cities, and religions, or with the institutions in which they work. However, their most rewarding compensation is found in family, which they sometimes worship and in which they find an alternative way of belonging and living within a tradition of their own.

General Characteristics

As small children, we are all first-chakra types. In childhood, we enjoy a sense of belonging to a greater collective—from family gatherings, to church rituals, to identifying with our national anthem and flag. We are also first-chakra types when we return home after a long day and feel the warm and sweet sensation of relaxing in our own place with our dear ones, interacting with our children, pets, partners, or friends. Even on a good day, we are grateful to return home and spend time with those to whom we feel we naturally belong. We find comfort in the routines of the home, like watching TV with our family at the exact same hour every day.

Whether we like it or not, we all tend to develop a first-type perspective and first-type qualities from around the age of thirty-five on. We begin to become more realistic and grounded as we establish our way of life, develop personal connections, and define our aims. The more we age, the deeper our commitment to certain frameworks like work and family becomes. We aspire to attain a steady income and surround ourselves with more or less the same friends. We cultivate a set of good and bad habits, and establish rituals in our lives. We become more set in our ways and become known to others as a clearly defined personality.

While we obviously pay a heavy price for this rather predictable and unexciting life, we also gain the healthy sense of being deeply rooted in our surroundings. The sense of many possibilities that perhaps filled us in younger years diminishes, but it is replaced by the feeling that this is, in a way, what life is all about.

In childhood, our parents usually embody first-chakra values for us. They tell us, much to our annoyance, that we should prepare for the future and think long-term; we should make careful and responsible choices, and become respectable figures in society. When we are older, we sometimes surprise ourselves by telling our children the same things.

First-chakra qualities are often likened to the heaviness of the elephant. Yogic scriptures also equate this type with the ant. This is perhaps the best metaphor for this personality, since it captures the hardworking and labor-loving nature of the type. Ants share the enthusiasm of Builders. They find great purpose in working to sustain their colony. They tirelessly carry grains and any other pieces of just about anything, battling any obstacles in their way to further their great communal project. Of course, any such construction demands endless repetition and a process full of near-ritualistic routine. But when you are gifted, like first-chakra types, with a worldview made up of cycles and continuity, you find beauty in this unwavering repetitive effort. Builders don't hope that, one day, their labors will end, because they deeply believe in the value of work and building.

Builders are not ambitious, however. They don't aim at the heights of life, since they are more interested in deepening their roots. Instead of ambition, they cultivate a great diligence. And sometimes, diligent people who love to strive for better results are more successful than those who are ambitious, yet less meticulous. Builders may not seek advancement or recognition for themselves, but they are highly productive, which makes them beneficial and truly indispensable for human society. Humanity literally relies on them. And since they are reliable, their shoulders are generally broad enough to accept the burden.

While most other types are easily bored by small details, this type's motto is, "God is in the details." Indeed, they have a great passion for details, even ones that strike others as utterly negligible. They find it pleasurable and meaningful to attend to these details, especially when other types abandon them in despair. In general, other chakra types watch Builders with amazement, wondering how they can speak passionately for hours about tiny details and how they can dedicate their entire energy to ensure that everything falls into place. First-chakra types are capable of patiently following and studying a system without getting tired, and they can become deeply involved in processes that don't lead to any thrilling climax.

This love of steadiness and stability keeps them closely tied to the warmth and security of their homes. They are intensely family-oriented, and their sense of family and of home are usually tightly integrated. Renting a flat will not suffice, and they are not the type for fleeting engagements. Rather, they will aspire to a home that will belong to them and their progeny. This may even extend to a desire for a land of their own. Anything that feels as if it could extend to infinity feels more proper and worthy to them.

This type's connection to the land—to homeland, house, and territory—is as deep as it can be. They are almost always attached to a place; if they are driven from that place for some reason, they become very nostalgic about it. They are content to live in one place forever, without the nagging longing that other types experience for "moving on" and trying other homes or other places. First-type philosopher Immanuel Kant, for instance, never traveled more than 10 miles from Konigsberg during his whole life.

Builders don't like going on adventures and are reluctant to undergo extreme changes in their lives. They actually wish for just the opposite—that everything will remain solid and steady and that life will be as undramatic as possible. That is why they are also financially conservative and shy away from making risky decisions. They tend to build toward a future of security.

Builders are not experimentalists at all. If they are religious or spiritual, they tend toward established religions and traditions with a long history behind them—Buddhism, Christianity, or other systems that are institutionalized and have a fixed dogma. They are comforted by prayers or meditations that have been used in exactly the same way for thousands of years. They view long traditions as being deeply rooted, and therefore, respectable—another virtue they value highly.

For this reason, first-chakra types don't like innovation—at least not those that come as a tremendous shock. It is not that they are disinterested in technology. It's just that they cannot bear anything that shakes up their lives. They tend to appear in historical anecdotes about science or culture as those who immediately reject any new discovery or idea. They compare everything that comes along to their traditional thoughts and beliefs. Anything that contradicts that tradition can't be right. They prefer slow change, and are suspicious of new possibilities. They may, however, put an innovation to the test and, after a few years of meticulous examination, they may let it gently infiltrate their system.

Because they are keen admirers of laws, Builders are readily obedient to them and happy when others obey them as well. This brings about a general air of respect and honor, which they deeply cherish. As highly moral beings, first-chakra types also appreciate manners and polite gestures. They feel that the more people treat each other kindly and with courtesy, the more they can connect to the inherent beauty of a higher order.

Since Builders live to build, they also love joining greater collective organizations to build with others. They are not individualists and always look for structures of which they can be a part—families, communities, nations, and religions. That is why they are also the greatest preservers of heritage and guardians of the wisdom, knowledge, and achievement of ancestors. They preserve their own family heritage, as well as national and religious traditions. They enjoy the sense of having a past on which their current life is built, and they feel that their ancestors are with them in spirit. They may grow nostalgic, claiming that, in the past, "everything was better."

Their search for security and stability drives first-chakra types to be communal beings who enjoy functioning and living within the framework of a larger group. If, on the other hand, they find themselves compelled to live apart from their familiar surroundings, or if they need to share their lives with some unsettling type, they may begin to feel unwell.

When thrust into an unstable or changing environment, they may even start to develop psychosomatic illnesses. They are thrown off-balance when faced with deep change or with more than one change at a time. They need to keep their routines intact. They also begin to crack when pressured and pushed to achieve.

Strengths and Gifts

Because they deeply appreciate long processes, Builders have a great advantage in relationships and partnerships. They are deeply loyal and trustworthy. On the other hand, they are by no means exciting lovers, and anyone looking for a thrilling love life should not expect that from them. What greatly compensates for the absence of excitement, however, is the steadiness they bring into their relationships, making others feel that they will always find the same person every day. Since they are faithful, they find it quite easy to commit to a relationship for life, and they are profoundly satisfied with the experience of marriage and parenthood.

Another beautiful trait of first-chakra types is their extraordinary patience. Unlike other types, they are gifted with an ability to delay gratification. They trust only long and gradual processes, so this quality comes naturally to them. They will avoid quick fixes and promises of immediate results in favor of efforts that are systematic and more reliable. This makes them a valuable support when friends and dear ones must endure some challenging long-term problem. Because they are generally gentle and relaxed, their presence bestows on those around them a sense of peace. They are good balancers for nervous and fiery people.

Builders are also endowed with a supreme practical intelligence, thanks to their combined traits of attention to detail, diligence, and mechanical understanding.

Challenges

First-chakra types are far from fiery. In fact, they actually tend to dullness and sometimes even apathy and lethargy. This is where the line separating relaxation and slowness from over-relaxation becomes unclear. Their balance can quickly turn into "over-balance"—for instance, waking up at the same time for thirty years, or working regularly in the same workplace for decades, or taking their rest at the same hour every day, or spending weekends more or less in the same way over a long period. These entrenched habits can make this type age more rapidly than others, since they do not naturally rejuvenate through change. In a way, they seem to like growing old.

Builders rarely experience extreme moods or states of minds; they are seldom extremely happy or extremely sad. They are stable—almost eternally "okay"—and therefore quite unexciting to be with. If they evidence any play of extremes, it is probably an alternation between lethargy and diligence. They can be very persistent over time, but then they can also slow down, as their kapha tendency makes them sink. This sinking tendency is what makes them prone to exhaustion, overweight, slow digestion, constipation, or physical inflexibility and blood stagnation.

First-chakra types are attached to food, less as pleasure and more because of its grounding and filling effect. In general, they are attached to possessions and are anxious when they sense that any of them may be taken away. They are also deeply attached to the past and tend to get stuck in it. Their possessiveness—not only to material objects but also to family, territory, and nation—can even turn aggressive, becoming almost an animalistic instinct to protect. Due to their identification with a core group, like family or nation, they find it easy to remain within a closed circle and ignore all others.

This type's most persistent negative emotion is worry, which can even escalate into anxiety. Because their experience in life depends on feeling solid ground beneath their feet, when things get out of hand, they can lose balance. They become quickly irritated when they feel that their structures are even a little threatened. They are also deeply troubled by thoughts about future stability.

Builders don't tend to have a great sense of humor and are definitely not funny people. They can easily become overly serious and even rigid, following rules, habits, and rituals of a moral code that they expect others to obey as well. For them, there is a "right way" to do everything—usually the way they have adopted from some conventional or accepted way of behaving. They barely tolerate unfamiliar modes of being. Due to the way they associate "law" with harmony, they may blindly follow laws and fail to question even nonsensical orders. This puts them at risk of obeying vicious laws just because of their respect for hierarchy and authority.

This type's attachment to the familiar can keep them in very unhappy circumstances—a failing marriage or a distressing work situation—without any hope of change. In this, they are sometimes almost deterministic, accepting their reality as if there were really no other choice. Yet beneath the surface, they simply fear change. Their diligence and love of details allow them to get caught in trivialities easily, firmly believing that this is what life is all about. This can entrap them in a one-dimensional and gray experience of the world.

One of the greatest challenges for this type is the tendency to live *for* their structures. In the same way that the order of things gets twisted when we "live to eat" or "live to work," they may immerse themselves in efforts to prepare a perfect ground, while not taking time to enjoy their actual lives. If all you live for is to keep your family safe, to make your house livable, or to ensure that the future is secure, what is the point?

Shadow Self

Builders don't like change. It is as if they simply don't understand why the divine or the higher reality would create a changing world when it could have created stable and unchanging forms that would last forever. They want reality to be eternally stable, fixed, and repetitive. When a change in their reality takes place, they freeze—almost like an animal caught in the headlights of an approaching vehicle. This is why I call their shadow self the "frozen self."

Builders feel safest when dealing with details. They cling to details as much as possible, because they make them feel grounded. They also cling to their sense of belonging to certain solid structures, like family, institutions, or religions. They basically fight all their lives against life, trying to prevent change. Death, for them, is the ultimate change. They simply don't know what to do with it. This struggle makes them develop a certain way of coping with weakness—a form of revenge against life. "If life is changing, at least I will not change; I will freeze." If they can't fully control life, at least they can fully control themselves.

For this, they create a heavily patterned and programmed personality that is not only their constitution, but also their own self-made creation based on the only way they know how to win in their fight against life. When they freeze, first-chakra types ground themselves so much that they can no longer move and become immune to any impression. They minimize their emotions, feelings, and experiences, and suppress everything in both their outer and inner experiences. Of course, they are very proud of being grounded in this way. They feel that their capacity to handle life like this is a highly desirable quality, while, at least in part, it is really just a form of anxiety.

The psychological work of the first type is to learn how to distinguish change from danger. For the most part, change is not dangerous. But recognizing this fact—which is obvious to other types—requires tremendous work on their part. They must learn not to freeze by admitting that they actually can change themselves and that they are not really happy with an unchanging reality.

They also need to stop clinging to details and realize that details are, more often than not, a form of safety net. It is good to know how to deal with details, but that doesn't mean that you should smother your world with endless small pieces of information.

Higher Potential and Destiny

Coming from the realm of universal law and order, where laws govern the universe and maintain everything in peace, Builders are our teachers for a right way of living. They lead us to a path of balance and health, reminding us that without a safe ground, no healthy life can ever flourish. They hand us a roadmap to a wholesome and ethical society, and show us individual ways to maintain a life that is aligned with planetary and cosmic rhythms. They reveal to us the hidden laws that keep our bodies, minds, relationships, and communities in a state of lasting peace and harmony.

In the presence of a first-chakra type, we feel calmer. They give us a sense of anchoring and stability, as they are connected to the basic sanity of a greater order. They teach us the great importance of stable structures like wisely planned schedules and a steady income. These structures are like channels and containers through which everything in our lives can flow with ease. They not only fill us with a basic sense of security but also make us feel healthier. Life can seem so messy at times. But when it is supported by structures, we can withstand any turbulence.

Builders show us the importance of inner and outer order as an expression of perfection and harmony. And they show us that we have a deep need for this order. Just think how much more relaxed our minds, emotions, and bodies could be if we put our lives in order. Since life is by nature disruptive, the least we can do is to put everything that is under our responsibility into order. By achieving order in our lives, we can also attain self-mastery. Seen from this perspective, structures and order are not only functional but also spiritual.

Builders encourage us to appreciate small details. As nagging as they may seem, details add beauty to life and support it. When your house is clean, it creates room for a more harmonious life. Moreover, many small details, when neglected, tend to grow into huge problems. One structure we are particularly reminded to take care of is our physical bodies, which require a healthy routine, nourishment, and calm. The reality is simple: when our bodies grow weak, it doesn't matter how great our ambitions may be. Our physical problems will chase after us wherever we go and thwart those ambitions.

Builders show us the beauty and joy of routine, which can connect us to a sense of cyclical rhythm. While routine may seem boring and something we crave to escape, in reality, it is vital. Do you really want to have to invent your day every morning? To rethink your life over and over again?

Builders also encourage us to overcome laziness and to cultivate diligence, love of effort, and patience as qualities that will bring lasting results in our lives. Moreover, they remind us that this love of effort is not only for our own benefit, since our efforts—just like anyone else's—are in service to the community and to the world at large. Even our need for money, which we may sometimes complain about, leads us to look for ways to serve our community.

One of the major gifts of this type is to show us the importance of community in general, and the role of the individual in interaction with a greater whole. They awaken in us the longing for a community founded on ethical relations with virtues like respect, justice, honor, and righteousness as our guiding light. They show us the value of self-restraint in establishing social stability and bring us back to the values of traditional society—self-dignity, humility, respect, loyalty, and a reverence for a healthy hierarchy.

This type can awaken in us a love of cycles and connection to greater cycles of life through the beauty of rituals and customs. There are important cycles in our lives as well as in natural processes and, whenever we perform a ritual or a ceremony, we are able to pause and feel more connected to the greater rhythms that are found in the land, on the planet, and even in the cosmos.

Builders remind us to honor our roots. They teach respect for the family that gave birth to us, for the state that is our larger community, and for the land that gives us sustenance and support. In general, they teach us that honoring all visible and invisible structures that hold us can only benefit and strengthen us. There is beauty in connecting to the land, including the joy of returning to the same lakes, trees, houses, and relatives. They also show us the significance of connecting to the past—including the deep past. Though the pace of life today is accelerating rapidly and we often feel that only progress counts, we still derive power from preserving past traditions, ancient wisdom, and the accumulated learning of the ages.

Achieving Balance

There are several lifestyle changes that first-chakra types can make to balance the excesses in their constitution.

» Avoid resting too much. Resist the temptation to fall asleep at midday. While this may seem refreshing, it may make it hard to get started again, since this practice increases the kapha element.

» Color your routine with some quick movement or action. For example, try five minutes of meditation or some physical activity after one hour of work. This can prevent you from sinking too deeply into one ongoing activity. Listen to some invigorating music from time to time—not classical or heavily patterned music, but pieces that cheer you up and keep you elevated.

» Introduce some dynamic physical activity into each day, like yoga or aerobics.

» Every now and then, go on an "intentional adventure" that deliberately breaks your routine or evokes excitement. Adventures and wisely used leisure can remind you that, within the continuum of time, there is not only past and future, but also the present.

» Develop a level of detachment that will help you realize that life's structures are just meant to enable something else, not serve as the purpose of life itself. Family, for example, is not the purpose of life, but rather a support to make you feel safe so you can do other things.

» Develop ways to step outside your core group—home, family, community, or nation. One way to do this is by serving a greater cause. Look for systems that are truly worthy of your efforts and devoted to lasting and noble purposes and values. This will keep you from getting stuck in small details that don't relate to a broader context.

» Spend time in the company of lighthearted and wakeful people. Being only or mainly in the presence of your own type can greatly enhance your excessive tendencies, like sluggishness, over-seriousness, and obsession with trivialities.

Finding Fulfillment

There are several paths first-chakra types can follow to fulfill the potential of their constitution.

- » Enjoy your peaceful routine, your stable lifestyle, and your solid structures without making excuses. Appreciate your strengths and aspire to a life that is an ongoing process of building.

- » Ask yourself whether you are overly influenced by family members and friends who belong to a different type and who may try to persuade you to be more "adventurous." While this may be useful for restoring balance from time to time, make sure that this advice is not grounded in resentment of your nature.

- » Instead of questioning your attraction to structure, ask yourself what kind of structures make you happiest. Don't cling to any structure that doesn't work well just because it is the most familiar choice. Look instead for the most fitting one.

- » Make sure you are not swept up in today's tendency to look for self-employment outside established structures. This may put you under severe stress. If you want to engage in something less organized, look for work that is guided by a natural-born entrepreneur.

- » Acquire established and practical knowledge that is part of a known system. Institutionalized knowledge contains a vast range of information and wisdom that you can use to structure your life.

» Make sure you have a steady income. Financial risk and periods of time with no income are not wise for you at all.

» Seek out and stay involved with creating and supporting collective structures. Assume a role that lets you prepare the ground for some initiative, or define rules and codes of behavior and interaction, or arrange work processes for others.

» Choose a spiritual path that involves *pranic* practices or life-force–enhancing exercises. Activities like breathing exercises, Tai Chi, Chi Qong, fasting, or kundalini practices will encourage a pulsating energy to flow through you to counteract your constitutional solidity.

» Seek out a supportive spiritual community; don't be a loner. Choose an orderly spiritual path that is already established and well paved, since this type of connection to a lineage or a long chain of past practitioners will calm you. On the other hand, ensure that your path remains fiery enough to encourage some leaps of self-transcendence. Going on retreats every now and then to enhance your spirituality may give you opportunities for making such leaps.

Are You a First-Chakra Personality?

This self-test will help you evaluate the percentage of the first-chakra type's presence in you. Let this moment of self-evaluation be relaxed and playful. Try not to evaluate the presence of this type in relation to other types. Just consider how much you recognize first-chakra characteristics in your way of being, your perception of the world, and your natural and immediate inclinations. Do not try to make an intellectual judgment. Trust that something in you will effortlessly recognize itself.

If you have trouble assigning a percentage to this chakra, read each of the following statements and consider how closely you identify with them. If all your answers are 1s, you probably identify closely with the type. If all your answers are 4s, you probably don't. Use your responses to guide you in evaluating whether you belong to this type. Once you have assigned a percentage, write it down so you can compare it with your other self-evaluations. This will help you determine your three-part personality type.

» The world is an opportunity for building something solid—diligently and patiently establishing stability, ground, and peace of mind.

1. Greatly identify

2. Moderately identify

3. Loosely identify

4. Cannot identify at all

» I love dealing with details—calculations and figures, materials and accurate planning, pieces of information and schedules.

1. Very much

2. Quite a lot

3. Perhaps a little

4. Not at all

» An ongoing fixed and highly predictable daily regimen calms me greatly and fills me with a sense of harmony. I like this repetition, and when it is disrupted, I am quite unwell.

   1. Exactly how I feel

   2. Quite true

   3. Somewhat true

   4. Not at all true

» I shift from diligence and self-discipline to tiredness and dullness, and the other way around, quite often.

   1. True, on a daily basis

   2. Quite true

   3. Rarely

   4. Never

» I love being a part of a larger unit like a tradition, a family, a community, or a nation. It feels healthy and supportive.

   1. A significant component of my well-being

   2. Quite true

   3. Only to a certain degree

   4. Not at all

CHAPTER 2

SECOND CHAKRA

The Artists

The Artists

» *Presence in world population:* around 7 percent

» *Public domain:* recreation and entertainment, festivals and celebrations, art and nature

» *Typically found among:* musicians, artists, comedians, stage performers, dancers, clothes designers, tour guides

» *Dosha constitution:* pitta/vata (fire/air)

» *Dominated by:* the feeling center, impulse, senses

» *Shadow self:* the butterfly that gives nothing

» *Time zone:* this moment

» *Traditional animal:* butterfly

» *Famous figures:* Sappho, Van Gogh, Arthur Rimbaud, Rainer Maria Rilke, Yves Klein, Frida Kahlo, Oscar Wilde, Seraphine Louis, Andy Kaufman, Jim Morrison, Jim Carrey, Roberto Benigni, Will Ferrell, Rudolf Nureyev, Jimi Hendrix, Janis Joplin, Kurt Cobain, Amy Winehouse, Iris Apfel

It seems like a cosmic joke that immediately after the first-chakra type, the second type appears. A more just cosmic order would place the third type next, since both share some essential characteristics. Builders and Achievers are time-driven. Artists, on the other hand, live in the moment itself, with no purpose, no future, and no worries. They live for the sheer pleasure found in the here and now.

Yet there may be a certain logic to this. Second-chakra types have a tendency to be surprising and to do the unexpected. They can even be disruptive at times. Indeed, Artists are sometimes so out of order that other types are easily annoyed by them. They don't obey the common law and strongly resist conforming to it. Thus, finding the most colorful of all seven types smilingly sandwiched between the very serious first and third types may make sense. So forget about Confucius and the Ten Commandments. Now it is time to break the law.

Essence

The second chakra is located in the pubic area between the genitals and the naval. It holds within it the essence of impulse. Think for a moment of impulses you feel—times when you suddenly "feel like" doing something, when you feel urged to act spontaneously. Sometimes you may even surprise yourself with an uncharacteristic behavior or a wish that is not typical for you. For a moment, try to get in touch with the place from which all your impulses and cravings arise. This is the second chakra.

There, you will find the force in the cosmos and life that releases sudden changes, eruptions, and quick movements. This force is most simply known through the intense urges of desire and sexuality. More broadly, however, it includes everything in the cosmos that is unexpected, volcanic, and stormy. It is felt as an element that enters a system—sometimes your own—and causes disorder. But by doing so, it brings something new to life.

Think of it. Even the appearance of life itself was a sort of twist in the cosmic drama. At first, the universe consisted only of meteorites, planets, and rocks. Then—*suddenly*—lizards, giraffes, and hippos began to take form, many of them rather strange and some even funny-looking. With the passage of time (and for no apparent reason), new species—colorful, unique, and sometimes astoundingly beautiful—came on the planetary stage.

You can sense this same burst of life in yourself when you are overwhelmed by uncontrolled cravings, or when a poem or a melody forms in your head, or when you fall in love when you least expect it. You sense it whenever the basic colors of life's routines are brightened by stronger colors of excitement and thrill, whenever life's plain tastes are mixed with sharp and intense sweetness or spiciness, whenever life's ordinary feelings are overpowered by sensuality or ecstasy. Some, however, may not even be able to differentiate between feelings, emotions, and sensations.

These urges, which the dictionary defines as something between "bodily consciousness" and "appreciative or responsive awareness," seem to disappear as quickly as they erupt, and with the same intensity. Like butterflies, they emerge with magnificent colors, joyfully flutter around your garden flowers—and then quickly die. Like spring flowers, they fill the earth with vibrant beauty—and then disappear. This is the essence of the second chakra—this flash of creative thrill that makes you feel so strongly alive, but then disappears without leaving a trace. Where did it come from? Where has it gone? This world of impulses and feelings is a strange one indeed. And it is the world from which the second-chakra type originates. Luckily, we have the Artists to guide us through this subtle world of spontaneous feelings.

Constitution

Now imagine this world of impulse and feeling manifested in a person, with all its essential elements—the dominance of impulse, the eruptive and stormy nature, the sensual tendencies, the deep passions, and the restlessness. In the Ayurvedic system, the constitution of this person would be a mix of pitta and vata, of fire and air. At its core, this personality is fiery, passionate, and explosive—but not with the strongly burning fire of the third type. This is more like a flare—a brief burst of bright flame that burns with a sudden intensity, then quickly disappears. It is the vata (air) element that adds this quickness, this lightness, and an ever-changing structure.

The combination of pitta and vata endows second-chakra personalities with an intense appearance and, at the same time, one that is quite airy. This type is usually quite thin, not because they don't take pleasure in food, but because their constitution keeps them too quick and fiery to become heavy. While first-chakra types walk slowly and move heavily, second-chakra types walk in a passionate manner and move rapidly, as if they are flying around. They are extremely physical; it is apparent to everyone that they are very much "in their bodies" and enjoy being there. They love touching, hugging, and caressing, and always look for chances to do that.

The general impression given by second-chakra types is that they are "all over the place." When they enter a room, they storm into it, often scattering everything they carry with them and letting everyone know and feel that they are "here." They are very wakeful and outgoing, and are easily recognizable by their large, intense, and wide-open eyes.

Sphere of Influence

Artists do not make up a large proportion of the world's population—only around 7 percent. They act like the spice of human existence—and for good reason. If our world and culture were governed by them, we'd all be living in the here and now, enjoying everything and breathing life into our lungs, refusing to work too much, and only waking up at noon. This may not be a great recipe for a functional society, but it would lead to a much more joyful one.

I'm not talking about just poets, musicians, and singers. The term "artist," here, indicates a general perspective on life. It describes someone who sees life as art, as a canvas on which the interplay of colors, sounds, and textures creates a platform for an endless array of possible feelings and experiences.

The Artists' wish for heightened feelings leads them to seek extraordinary experiences, which makes them quite adventurous. For example, this type often engages in extreme sports. Unlike third-chakra types, who may engage in risky activities because of a desire to win medals or to be considered the best in their field, the second type does so because they love living on the edge, teasing death, and feeling more alive. Some of them even die in the attempt, but they don't seem to mind risking death. They are simply driven by an impulse that tells them they "must" do it.

They may jump from an airplane at a high altitude just to defy the laws of nature or to see how it feels to be a bird or a rocket. Austrian skydiver Felix Baumgartner, famously hailed as the "daredevil who free-falls from space," free-fell twenty-three miles to earth in 2012, traveling faster than the speed of sound. He told the British *Daily Mail,* "When you depressurize the capsule you think, 'This is serious now.' You can feel in your stomach and every part of your body that it does not want to be there. But," he added, "the view was amazing."

Second-chakra types are like sprinters, rather than marathon runners. They don't have much energy for long-lasting processes, because they get bored easily. Their mind-set hardly contains the perception of a future, so they are unable to conceive of ongoing or long-term activities. They only engage in quick projects and endeavors. That is why they can write good poems, compose beautiful melodies, and create impressive paintings on impulse. They excel at activities that are short and intense. But when things get too demanding, they simply lose interest. The joy they take in being creative is closely related to a feeling that they are a part of the celebration of life. While there are second types who were notable musicians or painters with relatively coherent and long-lasting careers, even these figures exhibit a mixture of commitment to process and an aversion to anything that builds too seriously toward a future.

Indeed, the butterfly element is too strong in some Artists. The infamous Twenty-Seven Club consists of musicians (rock stars in particular), artists, and actors who seem to share an auto-destructive impulse that leads to death at the very young age of twenty-seven. The unfortunate list of members is rather long, including Jimi Hendrix, Janis Joplin, Jim Morrison, Kurt Cobain, and Amy Winehouse—all of whom are, without a doubt, second-chakra types. They enter the world like a flash of light, shake it up with their immense energies of youth and rebellion, and then burn themselves out like a fire that consumes itself—all in twenty-seven unforgettable years.

Needless to say, not all second-chakra personalities end up so tragically, but they do have the tendency not to be long-lived, and a large number of them burn out their vital energies at an early stage in life, as did French poet Arthur Rimbaud. Yet they don't seem to care much, because they approach death with fearlessness and curiosity. Death, to them, is almost like a peak experience. They seem to flirt with it and to have a near-fatal attraction for it.

Role in Human History

Historically, it is second-chakra types who bring the spirit of celebration to the world. At first, people gathered into tribes to have strong allies in their struggle for survival. Once they felt reasonably secure in their caves, however, it was the second-chakra types who suggested painting the walls. Once they learned how to use drums to warn each other of danger, it was second-chakra types who captured those rhythms and encouraged their fellow cave dwellers to dance, and sing, and play music. Thanks to them, an actual tribal consciousness emerged that celebrated life and elevated it to the next level. Then the discovery of psychoactive plants supported the development of magical thinking, turning nature from a perilous yet useful first-chakra space into a colorful stage that second-chakra types could populate with deities who interacted with the tribe and provided opportunities for worship, rituals, and celebrations.

Thanks to Artists, nature and life thus became a rich experience. They introduced fertility rites and seasonal celebrations. They also brought the thrill of storytelling to the tribal campfires, spinning tales that were sometimes frightening, sometimes instructive, and sometimes beautiful and imaginative stories about the source of creation. They ignited people's minds by conjuring vivid images in a language that had previously been used only for the sterile exchange of information.

As great sensualists, Artists brought an awareness of the joy of the physical body. First-chakra types have a sense of the physical only as it relates to cautious grounding. They don't enjoy being in the body and don't perceive it as a source of pleasure. Artists, on the other hand, are like little children in their approach to the body—the naked body in particular. They love feeling through it, shaking it in dance, and arousing it to connect and unify with Mother Earth.

Worldview

To second-chakra types, life is a play of energies. To them, the earth seems like a gigantic amusement park with many attractions and many opportunities to experiment. Not for them a cautious examination of the attractions, playing it safe and ensuring they make the "right choices." Rather, they seek to understand life by immersing themselves in it in the spirit of experimentation. They feel that, since life as a whole was designed *for* experience, then we, as human beings, must devour life, take in everything and "seize the day." To them, life is more a trip or a journey on which to collect moments of laughter and tears, thrills and disappointments, not a purposeful endeavor with a definite end result.

Second-chakra types don't take life too seriously. For them, life is a bit of a joke and God, if God exists at all, is kind of a joker. If there is such a thing as a divine will, it doesn't seem to them as if we were put here to work too hard, but rather to feel life and appreciate it. Otherwise, they argue, what is the point?

Artists are dominated by the feeling center, but they know that simply feeling life is not enough. They experience life intensely, feeling everything as strongly as possible—happiness and pleasure, but also pain. If you cry, they argue, do it fully, with all your might; make it a drama, a theater of tears and sadness! They are always on the hunt for new kinds of feelings and sensations outside the range of familiar human experience. They explore, not only the outside world but also the inner world of those elusive and fleeting substances called "feelings."

Artists seek out states of ecstasy. The word "ecstasy" derives from the ancient Greek word meaning "self-forgetfulness." To be ecstatic thus means to bring yourself to a state in which you lose yourself. To second-chakra types, this is where life begins. You don't just dance; you become the dance. You don't just sing; you become the song. You don't just have an orgasm; you become the orgasm. You lose yourself in the experience. Artists are endowed with a very high capacity for feeling. Feelings are about intensity, passion, energy, vitality, and totality. As experts in engaging in experience, they look with pity on those who struggle to feel fiery energies, experience overwhelming sensuality, and appreciate immense beauty.

You can recognize second-chakra types by their ability to experience things directly, explicitly, and physically. They love to show off. They are actors, after all. Remember the movie in which Harry and Sally are sitting in a restaurant arguing over whether women can convincingly fake orgasms? Sally—clearly a second-chakra type—makes her point by faking an orgasm so convincingly that all other diners are shocked into silence. Then a woman calls the waiter over and whispers, "I'll have what she is having." When a second-chakra type like Sally experiences something this strongly, others notice, thinking to themselves, "How is he/she doing that?"

The capacity of second-chakra types for direct experience influences and shapes their spirituality. But they won't be inhibited by conventional and introverted meditation postures. Their spiritual experience is all about fireworks and peak experiences. They want to explode in meditation. If they are religiously or spiritually inclined, God is not an abstract to them. God is nature and its forces; God is found in beauty, the depth of our senses, and the orgasmic explosion of the body. They feel most spiritual when they manage to make total use of their senses, when their senses are wide open to receive everything. Since they are not abstract or conceptual people, but lovers of life, they naturally find eternity within the world, in every flower and cloud. But they are lovers of freedom as well. So they find God in experiences of breaking barriers and limitations, and in moments when they feel that everything is possible and unconstrained.

Of course, as seekers of intense experiences who are mainly excited about being excited, the romantic approach of Artists is quite problematic. They are enthusiastic lovers, but they much prefer the initial stage of infatuation over the actual "love"—the gradual and often tiresome day-to-day building of a relationship. Even just hearing the word "relationship" may make them quite weary—such a long word, with so many syllables.

Artists, for better or worse, only feel alive when they have peak experiences and ultimate pleasures—when they manage to enjoy the best food, the best music, or the best landscape. They get bored easily when things stop stimulating their senses and conclude that life, real life, must be "elsewhere."

General Characteristics

As children, we all had the chance to be second-chakra types—crazy happy-crying toddlers who sob intensely because they just lost a balloon and, a second later, are amazingly happy because they get a new one. Second-chakra types never lose these childlike (but also childish) tendencies. In a way, they are, for better or worse, forever young, forever children.

Many of us were also second-chakra types when we were teen-agers—and perhaps some of us even in our twenties, when we were experimenting very intently with life's energies. We were adventurous and took risks, were extremely romantic—sometimes even in a "suicidal" and tormented way ("She left me! I want to die!"). Everything was magnified; everything was wonderful and terrible. With each instance of falling in love, it seemed as if the whole world was illuminated. Then, as love faded away, it seemed as if the whole world came apart. We were very moody, indulging in endless cycles of ups and downs, being angry and resentful, loving and joyful. And each changing mood felt so meaningful that we secretly enjoyed even our most terrible moments. Even a sad feeling, as long as it was brightly and intensely colored, brought a strange excitement.

Likewise, second-chakra personalities are constantly overly excited. In fact, they *need* to be excited. If they are not excited, they fear they may not be alive at all. This encourages them to react strongly to things, and that is why, to them, all experiences must be either horrible or wonderful. They are not content with any middle ground. They love being moody and don't really want to be balanced, because balanced, to them, means "dead." This is merely the Artist in them seeking to enhance and exaggerate the "drama."

This can easily annoy other types. When, for instance, this type listens to you, they give you the feeling that what you do is extremely exciting, even if you are describing a rather boring task. Their excitement is like a sun that shines on everything; wherever it shines, it brings light and warmth. Then it moves on and sheds its rays elsewhere. The memory of a second-chakra type is quite short-term. Unlike types that accumulate and store knowledge, they quickly forget, because they tend to live in the moment. Like butterflies, they are of the here and now, and their brains are designed for this. They are like children—cute, yet terribly irresponsible. Since they live in the moment, when things are terrible, they think, "That's it! It will be like this forever! It will never be fine again!" Then things change for the better, and they think, "That's it! Nothing will ever go wrong again!" They forget what troubled them a moment before, and only those who suffered with them while they were distressed remember.

Artists learn through the body, not through the mind. Even when they listen to an intellectual lecture, it is their body that is learning. They "feel" into things and hardly think. This enables them to appreciate high-quality materials, and they are prepared to spend a lot of money on beautiful clothes and objects. This tendency is supported by the fact that, as seekers of good feeling, they also look for comfort. They admire anything that is aesthetic with an extraordinary sensitivity—nature, a work of art, a piece of music—which also makes them highly poetic and artistically inspired. Sometimes, however, they may strike others as untidy or even unclean due to their restlessness and messiness.

Second-chakra types are always humorous and enjoy laughter. This includes having a healthy sense of irony that makes them able to laugh at themselves. This gift of lightness and laughter makes them very valuable to other chakra types. Almost all great comedians are second-chakra types. They do something for us that we don't know how to do ourselves. They can look at our overly serious world and see it as a funny and even ridiculous one. They immediately see the mess inside the order. Roberto Benigni's bittersweet *Life Is Beautiful* demonstrates this by depicting a father who kept his child's spirit up in a concentration camp by making fun of the horrific events that were taking place around them. Artists tend to recognize an aspect of the divine comedy that somehow balances our dramatic life. As Voltaire once wrote, "God is a comedian playing to an audience that is too afraid to laugh." But second-chakra types are not afraid to laugh. Instead, they help us release our tensions and see the ridiculousness of things.

Artists are also keen lovers of freedom. As such, they belong only to themselves and, like wild horses, are very hard to tame. They don't like structure, because they love change and a sense of independence. They also like breaking the law now and then for the same reason. Where a first-chakra type will obediently walk away from a Do Not Trespass sign, a second-chakra type will be intrigued by it and want to find out what is on the other side of it. Every now and then, they feel the need to do something naughty.

Second-chakra types are pleasure hunters and, in general, can be regarded as the greatest lovers of life. They are intensely passionate and want to celebrate life, squeezing every last drop out of it. They exhibit high levels of sensuality and eroticism, since they naturally possess a lot of burning energy in their genital region, where the second chakra is located. This makes them quite good lovers, and they are generally enthusiastic about sexuality. They are sometimes sexually unconventional and wild, taking less accepted sexual paths.

Many second-chakra types don't like mornings. They may wake up depressed and need time to enter the day. They simply don't like the feeling of routine, so they often feel much better in the afternoon and evening. They are quite often night owls. When they are completely unrestrained, they go to bed very late, after some clubbing and dancing and drinking, and sometimes wake up in the middle of the day. In general, they like celebration and parties, and are dancers at their core.

Artists are great travelers, especially when travel promises some uncharted adventure. They dearly cherish the feeling that they are free to move from place to place, and they have an aversion to the idea of settling down too much. Second-chakra types always need some quick movement to disrupt what, to them, seems like a threat of stagnation, which they fear may strike at almost any given moment.

As parents, second-chakra types do not exhibit the same responsible patience that other parents naturally possess. Most certainly, they are not the thoughtful kind of parents you can approach for serious advice. However, they have one great advantage over other parents—their funny and childlike nature. This allows them to relate to a child's nature even during the agitated stage of adolescence. Because in many ways they never get old, they are fun parents to be with even when they are seventy.

Strengths and Gifts

Second-chakra types are quite fearless. They enjoy experimenting and are not afraid to take risks. They also show great flexibility at times of change and are prepared to leave the past behind and detach where others struggle to let go.

They are colorful, entertaining, and interesting beings. They find many things compelling. Their high level of natural joy, cheerfulness, and enthusiasm makes them attractive and easy to be around. They are easy to talk to. They can get really excited about what you say—even if, in five minutes, they won't remember what you said. They turn their natural reservoir of passion toward you and give you the feeling that you and they are the only people in the world. Since they know how to enjoy life, it can be a lot of fun to be in their company.

In addition, second-chakra types are sensitive to beauty and nature. They are endowed with a developed physical intelligence, which enables them to know what is right and what is wrong for them through the body. This intelligence imbues them with the capacity to feel as deeply as possible through their senses in a way that no other type can.

Challenges

Second-chakra types can be quite egotistical and, to a certain degree, even narcissistic. As far as they're concerned, everything, including other people, revolves around their feelings. How they feel is all-important, and the people around them are but an extension of their own excitement.

Artists can be intolerably intense. Although they are fun and light to be with, sometimes being around them can be just too much. They can be too excited, talkative, and quick for most other types, as if they are unable to control their excessive energy. Other types may just want them to slow down from time to time.

Second-chakra types can give you the fantastic feeling that you alone exist in the world. But don't forget that they give the exact same feeling to others as well. This can make them disappointing lovers, because, when the morning comes, you realize that you *were* the only one in their world. This can be maddening, because they do not experience continuity. When they say their love will last forever, it is real to them *at that moment*. They don't think about the future and so don't understand why you might feel betrayed. Because of this, they can be quite unstable in relationships. They like falling in love, but find it difficult to go deeply. Indeed, they are almost unable to understand a relationship that grows by overcoming obstacles. They don't recognize shared struggles as a form of love.

As charming performers who like to give a good show, Artists tend to feel as if they are on stage even in real life, and so are often not authentic. They can be impulsive and hasty, and this sometimes makes them unreliable. They follow one impulse after another. They know how to start things, but not how to complete them. They don't recognize that projects in real life demand perseverance after the initial excitement and inspiration fade away.

Moreover, they can burn themselves out energetically because of their hyperexcitement. They are prone to addictions and obsessions—sex, extreme sports, drugs, and more. They always want to have more of everything that gives a good feeling. Their overflowing energy often leads to unhealthy and decadent lifestyles, to overindulgence in pleasures like alcohol, smoking, clubbing, and to a disordered life structure in general. They are attracted to danger and can be self-destructive and outrageous, doing things that are unheard of and scandalous. This doesn't mean that they cannot restrain their impulses or overcome them. It just means that it requires more effort for them to find alternatives for all the feeling enhancers that attract them than it does for other types.

Second-chakra types can spend too much money, yet often tend to be lazier than other types. They dislike hard work and find it difficult to commit to projects and structures. They much prefer living in the possible, not in the actual.

Artists know how to enjoy, but they also know how to be depressed. When they sink, they really go into a free-fall. Depression, melancholy, and moodiness are very familiar to them. The problem is that they like the ups and downs; they don't really want to attain some plateau of relaxation. When this enters their relationships, they are sometimes argumentative, slamming doors and creating drama just to spice things up.

Second-chakra types take great pride in knowing better than anyone else how to live in the moment. Because they know pure enjoyment, they look down on others who don't. What they don't realize, however, is that they are letting real life slip through their fingers. After all, huge parts of life are revealed only if you commit, become serious, and build into the future.

Shadow Self

If there is one thing that Artists hate, it is effort. They are surely the laziest humans on earth, and in general they suffer from a Peter Pan syndrome—never wanting to grow up. That is why I call their shadow self "the butterfly that gives nothing." Even when they are fifty or sixty years old, they still want to be like small children, running around among the grown-ups who do all the work. Like little children, they just want to have fun and remain irresponsible, selfish, and deeply uncommitted. They even translate their laziness into a philosophy of life.

Second-chakra types only want pleasure and strongly resist experiencing pain. Pain is a strange phenomenon that they avoid at all costs, using the power of their compensatory mechanisms—strong feelings and excitement—to do so. They make sure that they feel excited and "great" all the time, and constantly try to elevate their spirits, convincing themselves that, truly, they are not feeling pain at all.

In reality, however, they live in tremendous fear—a deep dread that if they give themselves away to something, they will literally die. That is why they don't enter into anything too seriously, feeling that, if they do, it could be the end of their freedom and of themselves. So they spend their whole lives jumping from place to place, spreading charm and laughter, and trying to cover up their incompetence with beauty. This keeps everyone, including themselves, from noticing the reality—that behind their inability to sit still for more than a short period of time, there lurk huge fears and anxieties. They are afraid of life as a grown-up, a life in which they will one day have to build something. After all, structures mean not having options, and not having options is worse than death.

Their solution is to pretend to be grown-ups. They look like grown-ups; they do grown-up things. But it is all a façade. They also expect to enjoy all the benefits that only those who commit themselves can enjoy. But they give nothing. For example, they want to feel the depth of love while never making a commitment. Or they want to experience the fruits of hard labor while remaining lazy. They only want the fun parts of life, without the effort required to obtain and sustain them.

Artists cope with this weakness by dazzling everyone with their charm and enthusiasm, while inside they actually feel quite sad. They are "sad clowns." When the laughter fades, when they are in a dark room sitting by themselves, they feel a creeping sadness, which, of course, they cheerfully deny. They carry this sadness because they know, deep down, that they lead a meaningless life. Knowing that they cannot enjoy the meaning of life that others experience, they end up feeling that they can achieve nothing.

Artists forever postpone their lives. Life is always happening at some other time—"One day, I will do that." They constantly give excuses as to why "now" is not the right time for engagement. And they hope no one will notice that the "right time" never comes.

In fact, second-chakra types always hope no one will notice. For instance, they tell everyone that they love them, but they never really give their heart away. They don't know what it means to do so, because they enjoy the feeling of complete nonattachment and are truly proud of it. They value their ability to leave things behind and to completely forget about them. They interpret this as freedom, and even as a built-in form of spirituality and transcendence. Artists take pride in their freedom, seeing it as a way to compensate for other weaknesses. Any threat to their freedom is therefore very unsettling to them, because it diminishes their good feelings and causes them pain.

To curb their shadow self, Artists must learn to separate commitment from death. Commitment is not death, but meaning, and there is no meaning in life without commitment. They have to grow up, and that is quite a challenge for a Peter Pan. They must also learn how to accept pain and effort—not only how to encourage others to make an effort, but to actually do it themselves. Above all, this personality type must face the sadness inside them. To begin with, they need to admit that there even *is* such a thing as sadness and avoid constantly justifying their way of life. It is not society with its morality that bogs them down. It is an inner voice telling them that something is wrong—that they are, after all, missing something.

Higher Potential and Destiny

Second-chakra types teach us to awaken our numbed feeling center. Feelings are elusive and intangible to our rational minds, and we have difficulty clearly distinguishing them from our emotions. The feeling center is our excitement center—the place from which we derive our totality, intensity, passion, happiness, joy, and liveliness. Artists live in this center, so they naturally and contagiously radiate and transmit it.

Many books and films depict second-chakra types who enter an overly ordered world and fulfill their role by disrupting everything. In all of these creations, the representatives of the orderly world realize their unconscious need to experience a more complete life through this forgotten piece of their being. Nikos Kazantzakis's well-known book *Zorba the Greek*, which later became a movie under the same name, is a good example. The story features a young English author who comes to Crete for business and meets an exuberant second-chakra peasant named Zorba, who teaches him how to enjoy life even under the most trying circumstances.

For Artists to fulfill this higher role in the world, however, they must learn how to turn it into a service. They must transform their energy from an egotistical experience into an offering that can actually be transferred to others. This is perhaps their greatest task.

We all find a second-chakra type nagging from our lower belly when we are overly ambitious or overworked, or when we take things too seriously. We then hear a voice inside us that asks, "Is this really life? Am I missing something?" That is the voice of the second chakra speaking.

Second-chakra types represent the totality and passion that can fill us when we are eager to exhaust life's experiences, to feel life fully, as if we live only once and this is our chance. In the movie *Dead Poets Society*, an outrageous English teacher engages with high school boys from an elite conservative boarding school and shakes up their lives through poetry. His mantra is *Carpe diem* (Seize the day). This teacher is clearly a second-chakra type whose mission is to encourage his students to become intoxicated with life. For him, nothing less will do. We can never be reminded enough that life is exciting, adventurous, and full of possibility. Unfortunately, our habit of narrowing down and settling for less obscures this reality time and again.

Second-chakra types remind us of the intensity and the blessing of the moment. They show us that it is more than enough just to be, and that it is possible to connect to life at any given moment. Life is not measured only by whether or not we have achieved our goals. Life is, in a way, already complete and fulfilled, if we only make ourselves available to acknowledge this.

Appreciation is a beautiful quality of second-chakra types. Because they are less "busy," they are able to recognize beauty and to let it in. Just like children who still haven't lost their connection with the wonder of everyday details, the beauty that is right under their noses, this type possesses the capacity to widen their senses—and to remind us to do so as well. They are here to show us that we can jump into life at any stage, that it is never too late. This is the gift of eternal youth, to know that there is always an unaffected, smiling child in us, no matter how much we age or how serious we become.

Artists fill us with life's sweetness through music, comedy, poems, and paintings. They help us counteract all the bitter and sour tastes we experience throughout the day. At the same time, they add spice to life—like chocolate with chili—to remind us that life is both sweet and naughty. In this, they also hand us the gift of liberating humor and laughter as indispensable qualities that can soothe our overly serious souls.

Sometimes, this type can strike us—wrongly—as one-dimensional and superficial happy "clowns." In reality, however, they represent a profound philosophy that teaches us that our senses, perceptions, and experiences can take us so much deeper than mere enjoyment. Below the visible world, there is an ocean of feeling. In fact, we fulfill only a minute part of our ability to feel. Artists put us in touch with these feelings—some dark, as they come from the subconscious, some strange or shocking, and some unfathomable. Many great poets who stretched the limit of our feelings were second-chakra types.

Artists show us that a feeling that seems like a mere sensory reaction is actually divine. They are, for example, the source of the idea of sacred sexuality, which demonstrates that something that is so physical can become an intense transformation and awaken the spirit. They are able to go fully into pleasure rather than denying it, and thereby find transformation and expansion of consciousness. While we can all dance and enjoy some level of release, Artists dance in a way that takes them to heaven, to an ocean of bliss, and to transcendence.

Second-chakra types teach us how to embrace our natural energies and the joy of the physical body. They help us recognize our sexual potential, telling us that we shouldn't be too moral and rigid. After all, sometimes laws are there only to be broken. They show us how to merge with nature and with the richness of the earth. They encourage us to have a "poetic spirit," to appreciate beauty, good taste, and elegance—not only in cars and clothes, but also in the simplest, most taken-for-granted details of life.

Imagine a life without poets, comedians, and musicians. Or a life without celebrations, parties, wine, and chocolate. Or a life without art and with only soulless and functional architecture. Imagine a world in which everyone dresses only in gray and black. This is the world we would be trapped in without the bright colors this type brings us.

Achieving Balance

There are several lifestyle changes that second-chakra types can make to balance the excesses in their constitution.

» Use enhancing substances like drugs and alcohol in moderation and avoid too many enhancing experiences like sex and all-night dancing. The feeling that you have an endlessly flowing, superfluous energy can be misleading, and you must avoid burning yourself out.

» If you are already in the grip of some addictions or obsessions, go through a cleansing process to get rid of these tendencies, because they are just burning out your nerves. Try to find healthy alternatives to alcohol, drugs, and sex. Don't try to go "cold turkey." One path to ecstasy must be replaced by one that is deeper and more refined, not with routine. Try healthy alternatives like creative expression, some forms of spiritual trance, dancing, merging with nature, intense *prana* practices, or tantric practices that transform sexual energy. They can help you channel your energy while at the same time feeding your love of the senses.

» Make sure your lifestyle doesn't get out of hand, but remains somewhat relaxing and orderly. Resist the temptation to lead a life of chaos, which can stir up emotional storms. Have at least one thing in your life that doesn't change to reassure you that all is well.

» Don't be overcome by your egoistical tendencies. Find a way to provide service to the larger community in your life, a way to practice unconditional love and compassion. Learn how to translate your inner fire into gifts.

» Make at least one a long-term commitment in your life—a relationship, a child, a job, or a spiritual path. Take responsibility for something, although this may go against your intuitive way of living. Freedom is not just remaining forever uncommitted.

» Practice patience and develop at least one long-term plan. Try imagining yourself living to ninety to give yourself a reason to invest in a more relaxed life.

» Make sure you spend time with other types. Seek out some "responsible adult," someone who is wise and diligent. Remain cautious of the kind of person who tells you to be "serious" or opposes your natural energies. Associate with people who are supportive and empathic, and at the same time inspire you to be orderly and responsible.

» Strive for mental clarity and avoid getting swept away by currents of unclear feelings. Try meditating quietly, especially when you feel that you are too engaged in your "ups and downs" and need some emotional balance. Avoid ecstatic spirituality without any relaxation, as this can be unbalancing.

» Don't put off getting up in the morning, as lingering in bed can cause depression, or at least a slight melancholy. Avoid missing out on morning activities. Instead, try taking a rest in the middle of the day as a form of quick rejuvenation. Maintain a schedule—not one that is too tight and scary, just one that gives some general outline so you feel supported by a structure rather than being completely scattered.

Finding Fulfillment

Here are several paths second-chakra types can follow to fulfill their potential while still remaining true to their constitution. Just as it would be unreasonable to catch a bird and force it not to jump around, it is not wise to squeeze a second-chakra type into a rhythm of life that is too slow or constraining.

» Keep your body active. Going to the gym is probably not for you; you need much happier forms of workout. Try dancing for half an hour each day. Accept the restlessness and agitation in your body, but learn to express it in healthy ways so it doesn't build up and turn into agitation in your mind or even anger.

» Use beautiful music and dance to channel your energy. Music is the language of the soul, and sometimes merely playing it can align your system.

» Be careful not to submit yourself to a life of commitments and routines that can dry up your spirit. Routine family life or an all-consuming job is probably not for you. Find frameworks that respect your love of freedom and that allow for your love of life—frameworks that respect your need to feel free to leave.

» Choose a career that ensures your independence and gives you sufficient space for creativity and initiative. You need to know that you can bring up new ideas and introduce innovations—then let others pursue and construct them. Seek out and design surprising elements in your workplace; sprinkle new spices and colors over the existing framework.

» Look for opportunities in any field of art: poetry, painting, dancing, singing, composing, acting, filmmaking, comedy—anything that puts feelings and their free expression at the center. Clothing design may work well for you, as you love giving style and beauty to things.

» Try teaching others ways to engage their own bodies—Tantra, yoga, Tai Chi, dance, acrobatics. Seek out activities that can be connected to nature and adventure—like being a tour guide.

» Explore spiritual paths that lead to experiential explosion, not those that encourage moderation or self-restraint. Cultivate extreme experiences that bring you to know God or the inner self as an explosion of feeling—for instance, kundalini arousal, Tantra, trancelike and cathartic practices, ecstatic dancing, or dynamic meditation.

» Maintain a sense of drama in your life and your spiritual practices. Remain prepared to surrender completely to God or to life, and within that surrendering, keep your body fully engaged. Cultivate a path that is full of pathos and poetic and romantic feelings.

» Actively include your body and your senses in all you do. Maintain your sense of freedom on any path you choose and be sure that path justifies your love of life and the senses. It must be something that blesses life and proclaims that life is holy.

Are You a Second-Chakra Personality?

This self-test will help you evaluate the percentage of the second-chakra type's presence in you. Let this moment of self-evaluation be relaxed and playful. Try not to evaluate the presence of this type in relation to other types. Just consider how much you recognize second-chakra characteristics in your way of being, your perception of the world, and your natural and immediate inclinations. Do not try to make an intellectual judgment. Trust that something in you will effortlessly recognize itself.

If you have trouble assigning a percentage to this chakra, read each of the following statements and questions and consider how closely you identify with them. If all your answers are 1s, you probably identify closely with the type. If all your answers are 4s, you probably don't. Use your responses to guide you in your evaluation. Once you have assigned a percentage, write it down so you can compare it with your other self-evaluations. This will help you determine your three-part personality type.

» The world is a field of endless possible adventures and we are here to fully experience all of them and, hopefully, miss nothing.

   1. Greatly identify

   2. Moderately identify

   3. Loosely identify

   4. Cannot identify at all

» Are you considered jumpy, agitated, and restless by others?

   1. Very much so

   2. Quite often

3. Perhaps a little

4. Not at all

» What would you say is the most active part in you?

1. Body and feelings

2. Emotions

3. Will and ambition

4. Mind and intellect

» How much do you like long-term projects and lifetime commitments?

1. Not at all

2. Somewhat

3. Quite a lot

4. Definitely my style

» How much do you like change and mobility in life (as opposed to routine and permanence)?

1. I only ever feel alive in this way

2. Very much

3. Only every now and then

4. Not at all

THIRD CHAKRA

The Achievers

The Achievers

» *Presence in world population:* around 25 percent

» *Public domain:* any competitive arena, competitive sports, Wall Street, the army, gym, street fights

» *Typically found among:* warriors, soldiers, businessmen, mountain climbers, Olympic athletes, heavy metal bands, rappers, gangs, mafia

» *Dosha constitution:* pitta/kapha (fire/water)

» *Dominated by:* the willing center

» *Shadow self:* the failure-fearing doer

» *Time zone:* the future

» *Traditional animal:* ram, bear

» *Famous figures:* Alexander the Great, Pelopidas, Alcibiades, Leonidas of Sparta, Spartacus, Toyotomi Hideyoshi, Oda Nobunaga, Joan of Arc, Columbus, Marco Polo, William Wallace, Attila the Hun, Hannibal Barca, Richard the Lionheart, Genghis Khan, Percy Fawcett, Heinrich Harrer, Bruce Lee, Muhammed Ali, George Gurdjieff, Che Guevara, Lance Armstrong, Warren Buffett, Vladimir Putin, Donald Trump

Shifting from the juicy and life-loving character of the second-chakra type to the warrior-like personality of the third-chakra type demands a bit of mental gymnastics. It is not that there is no similarity at all between them. In fact, both are exploding with excited energy. It's just that, for Artists, that energy is without direction. For Achievers, it is fully and eternally directed. Indeed, in some ways, Achievers are an interesting hybrid of Builders and Artists—a surprising mix of impulsive craving and careful planning.

Achievers make use of the planet's energy resources for gaining power and achieving ends. Whereas the first type builds from the earth's materials, and the second creates out of them, the third type builds structures on them that reach for the highest goals imaginable.

Essence

The third chakra, located in the upper belly at the solar plexus, holds within it the essence of force and power. The solar plexus is, subtly speaking, the storehouse of energy with which we gather and direct our being toward any purposeful action. Unlike the second-chakra essence, this energy is not an impulse, a flash, or a sudden eruption. It is a determined and steady force.

Force means drive, and drive appears when energy in the cosmos becomes concentrated and directed. Think of it as the pointed tip of the arrow of the universe. The universe is full of drives, forces, and strong energies that seem to push against any resistance to overcome obstacles or apply counterpressure. These forces and drives all move in a forward or outward direction and are the impetus behind every wish to expand, grow, and achieve. They are the antithesis of any sense of limitation.

The same force that makes everything in the world and the cosmos march forward, expand, and grow pulsates within us all as well. In the world of physics, we call this gathered energy that wants to drive everything forward "force." In the human world we call it "will." In us, it is the drive to overcome difficulties despite all obstacles, and the commitment to remain faithful to our goals to grow and expand. Why? Simply because we feel we *must*. It is the element in our nature that makes us aspire to grow ever stronger and become ever greater. This is the force behind the Achievers.

Constitution

The third-chakra type is an interesting combination of pitta and kapha—fire and water. Pitta makes Achievers intensely fiery, energetic, restless, and ambitious. Kapha makes them resilient and solid and able to express an unwavering determination.

Achievers are energetic and strong, and look different from the slim and quick Artists. Their essential fiery nature is contained, however, within a grounded and even immovable presence. Their posture, which is decisive and resolute, reflects this well.

Achievers can sometimes be quite fatty, although this does not make them sluggish, as Builders can sometimes be. They are highly focused and always speak "to the point." They give the impression that they know what they want, even if they only seem to be making small talk. They always appear to have a reason to engage in communication, and do everything with focused intent. They never do anything simply for its own sake; their actions are always part of a larger plan. When conversing with them, you always feel as if you are just one more step on the way to their grand design.

Sphere of Influence

Artists are sprinters, but Achievers are marathon runners who steadily advance while keeping their eye on the prize. They are the ones who dream of climbing a mountain, not for the sake of the adventure, but because they want to reach the top. They want to stick their flag on the highest peak—preferably one that no one has reached before. They want to be in the *Guinness Book of World Records*. They want to achieve world fame and show everyone that they are "someone."

These strong and proudly willful individuals constitute 25 percent of the world's population. Their large numbers, combined with a most intense willpower, makes their presence in the world undeniable. Just as we need Builders to create the structures within which we live our lives, we need Achievers to push society forward toward progress. Builders put everything in place; Achievers look at their meticulous constructs and ask, "Nice, but what's next?"

The energy of the third-chakra type is the very energy that pushes the world forward. That is why we can find them throughout society and culture, sometimes as promoters of the ideas of others, and sometimes as tireless initiators of their own. They are warriors and martial artists who are highly attracted to competition, winning, and mastering their physical powers. For the same reason, they are often Olympic athletes, fascinated with the bodily experience yet intent on overcoming physical weakness and developing nearly superhuman powers—along the way, of course, gaining recognition for their remarkable achievements. In this respect, unlike the Artists, their bodies are merely a means to an end.

Athletes may be either second- or third-chakra types. What determines their type is their main drive. Do they excel in their sport for sheer love of physicality? Or are they more concerned with winning? Those who compete because they love the challenge and the tension between "what is" and what "could be" are definitely Achievers.

In general, Achievers are drawn to all types of competitive sport, because they are attracted to the thrill of competition and are driven to win. This drive is present, of course, in other endeavors; it is simply more overt in sports than it is in other fields, where competition and its rewards are often far subtler and more restrained. Wherever there is an opportunity for breaking a record or establishing a benchmark, that is where you will find this type, struggling with determination and tremendous energy to achieve the unachieved or even the unachievable.

It doesn't matter to this type whether the goal they pursue is negligible or lofty. If they are driven, they will follow through at all costs, including taking dangerous risks. Any goal that demands mastery and that astounds others is worthy of their ambition.

Third-chakra types are often yogis, shamans, and magicians who are keen on achieving supernatural powers. A yogi of the third type seeks to acquire wondrous capacities by mastering the body, mind, and matter. Shamans and magicians of this type enjoy controlling, commanding, and conjuring, levitating objects through the power of their intention, or telepathically reading other people's thoughts.

On the other hand, third types are often found among social and political rebels, revolutionaries, and protesters. They are drawn to rebellion as a call to battle, since wherever there is something to fight for, there is a chance of winning as well. Like Che Guevara, they are less concerned with forming ideologies, and more concerned with implementing ideas and working to make them take hold. As activists, they tend to work underground, are anti-institutional and angry, and are sometimes even violent rebels.

On the other hand, Achievers may also be tyrants and brutal dictators who exhibit uncontrolled bursts of power and coercion. You can also find them within gangs, mafia families, and organized crime syndicates—any groups that appreciate power and force as a common language and shared value. Third types also thrive in both the heavy metal and the rap genres of music. Because this music is filled with enraged energy and not really sure what to do with it, Achievers can channel their third-chakra energies through it and give them voice.

Achievers like winning wars and building empires. They are the "conquerors" of the world in any arena they enter. In the past, they have been imperialists and world explorers; today, they are corporate and capitalist moguls. They have moved into the financial markets and into the entrepreneurship of Wall Street and Silicon Valley. Because Western society offers fewer opportunities for physical warriors and territorial conquest, they have gradually "mutated," taking the form of leaders who strive to take over the world economically and build financial empires. They are conquerors at heart—never satisfied, forever working to grow bigger, sometimes even seeking to exert their influence outside the realm of planet earth.

Because their arena for expression has changed, these warriors now wear mainly business suits and work in subtler and more cunning ways to achieve their goals. Beneath the surface, however, they are still all about the survival of the fittest and hierarchies of power.

Role in Human History

Historically, Achievers were strong individuals who disengaged from the tribal consciousness, which mainly sought safety and calm, to lead an expansion of power and dominion. Unlike others, they clearly wanted more and initiated wars to acquire greater resources and expand their territories at the expense of other tribes. Slowly but surely, their tribes transformed into nations that possessed vast domains. Even that was not enough for the third-chakra type, however, and their incessant striving eventually led to Imperialism. Alexander the Great, an obvious third type who unabashedly worked to conquer the world, serves to this day as a most striking example of this type. In fact, Achievers are the embodiment of the mythic "hero" who bravely takes on the mission to fight for and save suffering humanity. Greek and Roman mythologies are replete with these heroes.

Third-chakra types showed humans how far they could travel—for the most part physically, but also mentally and emotionally. They were the world explorers who chased the dream of crossing oceans and mapping uncharted territories. They rejected any sense of limitation within one country or continent, and, although the risk was high, persevered and ultimately "conquered" the globe.

Achievers led crusades in support of their respective gods or kings. Unfortunately, they were also responsible for the Inquisition and other movements in human history that sought to make everyone adhere to a single ideology. For better or worse, they were the superb executors of the utopian visions of their charismatic leaders. Whatever dubious dream these leaders pursued, their fellow Achievers were sure to become enthusiastic and dynamic followers, winning wars, fomenting revolutions, and constructing new regimes in their name.

Worldview

For the third-chakra type, life in and of itself is never satisfying. Indeed, to them, it seems quite circular, repetitive, and undirected.

For them, life is just a starting point. It only becomes interesting—as well as organized, dynamic, and meaningful—when there is a glimmer of something new, something better, on the horizon.

For Achievers, life is potential. Through willpower and determination, they strive to realize this potential and make life into a "success story." It is in this striving—in this sense of external and internal overcoming—that third-chakra types find the highest value. They perceive the world as a ground for competition, where species, people, and ideas meet and struggle for dominance. The winner is the one who demonstrates the strongest capacities, the most fearless determination, and the highest ambitions. This winner, of course, "takes all."

Friedrich Nietzsche's *Will to Power* is a perfect depiction of the third type's worldview. Nietzsche envisioned everything as driven by the desire and struggle for self-expansion. From biological forces to the human psyche to cultural behavior, he considered this the element that gave shape to all possible processes in the universe. Indeed, to Nietzsche, the world as a whole was a world of power:

> A monster of energy, without beginning, without end, a firm, iron magnitude of force that does not grow bigger or smaller, that does not expend itself but only transforms itself; as a whole, of unalterable size. . . . A play of forces and waves of forces, at the same time one and many, increasing here and at the same time decreasing there; a sea of forces flowing and rushing together, eternally changing, eternally flooding back.

Achievers believe in the language of power and force, and perceive the world through its hierarchies, measuring and comparing and, in general, being keenly aware of the dramatic rise and fall of forces all around.

This world of power is full of challenges, which third types believe we must not avoid, but rather embrace as opportunities. They believe the very process of fighting toward a goal constitutes the meaning of life. Obstacles are merely invitations to overcome and prevail. It is in the moment of overcoming that they feel they have deeply contacted the meaning of life.

The true self of a third-chakra type is a warrior, a hero of its own drama. Their mission is to break the shackles and triumph over the weaknesses of the flesh or any seemingly overpowering element that threatens from within or without. Their worldview as a whole is a mythology of heroism. There can be no self-acceptance, because the self can only be real when it becomes worthy through accomplishment and struggle. For third types, grace is found in their own efforts—in what they do without waiting for or relying on anyone.

Third types seek experiences of confidence, power, control, and self-expansion that give them the empowering feeling of becoming more themselves. Their gaze is turned upward to unreachable heights and peaks. Since the purpose of life is to conquer that which is the highest imaginable, they find their happiness in worldwide recognition, in prestigious rewards or awards, in high status, or in anything that makes them outstanding and "special."

Love is just one more thing to conquer for third-chakra types, while death is just another obstacle to be overcome by technology or supernatural powers. They seek to immortalize themselves, however, by being remembered for their achievements. The spirituality of a third type is based in peak experiences and fireworks. They meet their "God" at the summits of achievement, overcoming, and victory, and in the power of all-encompassing presence. In general, their conception of God is literally the "Almighty"—a being of infinite power and energy.

General Characteristics

Many of us were third-chakra types during our teenage years, when we experienced the urge to define ourselves. This process of self-definition stands, of course, in strong opposition to all others. To be "you," you must not be "them." These "others" include parents and any other authority figures. The teenage years are a time of rebellion, stubbornness, and sometimes rage, followed by the near-romantic agony of feeling "misunderstood." By insisting on and declaring our will, we feel like ourselves. An intense individuation also takes place as we struggle to position ourselves in the social hierarchy, comparing, adjusting, and fighting to become popular, while at the same time remaining authentic.

We are all third-chakra types when we feel that we can fulfill much more of our dormant potential and reach greater heights in our lives—when we want to be recognized for some excellence or accomplishment. Sometimes, we feel driven toward a destination that our entire conditioned being tells us we are unable to achieve. Yet, determined to become the hero of our own story, we gather all our forces to stay committed to our goal and to combat all obstacles, including overcoming frailties within ourselves.

When we succeed through great discipline, we enjoy a third-type satisfaction. Achievers want to embrace difficult challenges and resolve to meet them with all their powers, rather than hiding away or giving in to debilitating emotions. Their battle cry is, "What does not kill us makes us stronger."

Third types are governed by the willing center and have a highly developed intelligence of the will. This gives them the capacity to focus unwaveringly on any target. They simply lock on to a target and then move tirelessly toward it, like battery-operated toys that attempt to march forward even when they hit a wall. As long as the goal remains before them, they keep trying to reach it and are too inflexible to redirect themselves. This is not necessarily a weakness, since they are equipped not only with a love of challenges, but also with endless energy. They are always busy, always running somewhere. They never have enough time and keep to a schedule so tight that they often divide it into fifteen-minute segments.

Achievers are intensely future-oriented. While Builders lean on the past and Artists playfully enjoy the present, the third type sees only the future. With their goal in mind, everything else becomes just an obstacle to be overcome. This unique goal-oriented constitution often prevents them from getting in touch with their feelings and the feelings of others. Third types treat others the same way they treat themselves—seeing their feelings merely as weaknesses to be overcome. For them, the will always takes precedence over feelings, urges, and instincts. This naturally endows them with great self-discipline, at least when it comes to harnessing their inner forces to achieve important goals.

Because they are obsessed with hierarchies of power, third types constantly compare themselves to others. They take great comfort in validating that they are better than others, and they become terribly anxious when they realize that the achievements or powers of some may exceed their own. As soon as they sense any schematic or hierarchy—whether in the sphere of finances or of spiritual evolution—they become intensely focused on knowing where they stand in that hierarchy and if any other individuals outrank them. They always want to be the most accomplished in their field and, even when they are quite successful, can end up feeling frustrated if they don't achieve excellence. They are keen on collecting others' "success stories" and believe they *must* have a success story as well. Above all, they dread failure and are unable to accept it, since, more than anything else, they hate any sense of humiliation.

Third types enjoy accumulating money and possessions. They are not necessarily passionate about these possessions, however.

Indeed, they may not even know who the famous artist is who painted the picture they just hung on their wall. They are driven by the goal of acquisition and conquest rather than any desire to appreciate the objects they acquire. While Builders simply want to have enough and are hesitant to take risks, Achievers want to have more and thrive on risk-taking. "Enough" is too mediocre a goal for them.

Achievers are deeply identified with doing. Their motto might be a paraphrase of Descartes: "I do, therefore I am." They don't "do," however, because they are passionate about perfecting small details and creating perfect conditions; they "do" because they hope to achieve something far greater. They are highly practical people in the sense that they don't have much time or patience for contemplation or discussion. They are naturally more inclined to be executors rather than planners. In general, when they go to work, they don't just set out to do well in their jobs; their warrior instinct tells them that they are going into battle.

Third-chakra types don't understand the language of feelings or abstractions. For them, inner content must always be translated into action. When faced with subjective feelings or thoughts, they impatiently ask, "So, what do you want to *do*?" They only understand attitudes that manifest in actions; you either act on what you believe in, or you don't really believe in it at all. They are never impressed by someone who says, "I feel it, but I cannot express it." They only care about ideas that become concrete and practical actions in the visible world. A clear trait of the third type is that they are explicit and straightforward in their communication. They are transparent and say what they want. They also let everyone know when they're angry.

Achievers like working deep into the night because it gives them even more time to pursue their goals. They are often sleepless, full of energy and will, and restless with anticipation to storm into the morning and return to full activity. Nights spent in sleep are nights wasted, frozen in an awkward position and not getting anywhere. Even when they do go to sleep, their inner engine is still working.

Strengths and Gifts

One of the greatest strengths of the Achievers is their exceptional determination. While other types may find this quality very difficult to develop, third-chakra types are endowed with it naturally and abundantly. They are gifted with what can be termed "strategic intelligence"—intelligence that knows how to set a goal and how to reach it step by step. As long-distance runners, they know how to direct their will and to fix it with an unwavering persistence. They almost always know what they want and exhibit great confidence that they will get it.

Achievers have an impressive capacity to overcome challenges and obstacles. You might even say that they like hardship. Although they hate being "losers," fear of failure never weakens their readiness to battle with problems head-on. When asked for advice, successful third-type figures often reply that their greatest key to success is their ability to reject failure and their willingness to fail over and over in pursuit of their goal. They say that those who succeed are simply the ones who failed but kept on fighting. This can be a useful trait for those who tread the spiritual path, because it helps them face difficulties and even intentionally submit themselves to adverse conditions in order to practice self-overcoming. With this self-discipline, they can develop spiritual qualities that require them to pass demanding tests.

Third personality types also possess a high capacity for handling crises and are efficient decision-makers. They know how to manage stress and can easily control their emotions and instincts. While Artists often imagine that the whole universe revolves around their bad or good feelings, Achievers always subordinate their feelings to their higher goals. They are probably the most active chakra personality type, and they usually enjoy an ongoing sense of power and energy that they derive not from their bodies, but from their willing center.

Challenges

The indifference of this chakra type to other people's feelings can cause suffering. But they most likely cannot understand this complaint, since, to them, it is only natural that everything (and everyone) should serve their will. As a result, they can be arrogant.

While they are gifted with patience that keeps them fixed on their goals, Achievers are utterly impatient toward other people's difficulties and any processes that seem to stretch on without end. Being very quick themselves, they cannot bear the thought of energy wasted. They are intense control freaks. That is why they get very angry—not just angry, but enraged—when things get out of hand and they need to face an obstacle, sometimes in the form of another person. When this happens, they tend to see that person as a hindrance and they react with rage in their attempt to remove it. They sometimes don't hesitate to step on others while climbing the ladder of success.

It is hard to relax in the presence of an Achiever. Their intensity and willfulness—especially when they take the form of barely concealed manipulative and cunning behavior—can be demanding. They see enemies everywhere. In fact, to them, an enemy is anyone who seems to thwart their mission. This is the remnant of the classical "warrior" inside them who is always ready to fight.

Achievers are highly individualistic and clearly want to be credited with their own individual triumphs. They are not great team players. When they do collaborate, it is only because they understand that they require other people to complete their mission. Their style of collaboration is more like that of the basketball player who knows that if he wants to win the game, he has to throw the ball to another player.

Achievers are often intensely materialistic and greedy. Their entire life experience can be narrowed down to ambition. They tend to focus on their goals as if possessed and can have trouble knowing when or how to stop. Ironically, third types are also very frustrated. Even when they do reach a goal, since their constitution is all about *wanting* to reach a goal, they immediately move on to the next one. This entraps them in a constant feeling that there is always something "more"—more success or more power—to be obtained. Third types are governed so strongly by their need to strive that they often end up stuck and unsure about which direction to take, eventually ending up trapped in their own energy and heat. This is why they often find it hard to sleep.

In the same way, Achievers can get lost in their overachieving spirit and their hunger for power. This makes it difficult for them to distinguish truly worthy destinations from lesser ones. To them, a goal is a goal; they may gather all their will and turn over the entire world around them only to achieve something utterly negligible.

Achievers can also risk turning into overachievers. Lance Armstrong is a striking example of this. To them, the means always serve the end. Therefore, any measure can be justified for the "noble" purpose of reaching the highest goal.

Because third-chakra types can be compulsive and obsessive, they tend to unhealthy lifestyles and are at risk for certain addictions. The result of being under constant pressure to perform can lead to minimal sleep, a diet of junk food, and addictions like sexual excess, pornography, stimulants, smoking, or gambling. Unlike Artists, however, they are less interested in the pleasure provided by enhancing experiences and substances, and are more in need of a release for all their accumulated fire within.

Third-chakra types are most challenged in their intimate relationships. While Artists are unstable yet good lovers and Builders are boring yet loyal and faithful partners, Achievers, by their very nature, give love secondary importance in their lives. On the one hand, they can be extremely possessive, angry, and controlling; on the other, they may never spend time with their partner because they think of it as a horrible waste of precious time—even if that partner is sitting in front of them crying. To them, there is a whole world to manage and it depends on them and them alone.

In extreme cases, the third personality may become a destructive and dangerous element in society. Sadly, the world has suffered from many excessive third-type figures who used the world for their own uncontrolled power trip rather than serving it for the greater good. Because these figures possessed high levels of energy and will, they could—and sometimes did—succeed in ruining the world.

Shadow Self

The main struggle for Achievers is that they are always trying to become "someone." What they fear most is failure. Indeed, failing is their nemesis. Because they only measure themselves by the standard of success and failure—according to the way they rank on the social ladder or in a hierarchy—they have a horror of being disrespected or unrecognized for their achievements. Indeed, their whole life depends on respect and recognition. This is why I call their shadow self "the failure-fearing doer."

Achievers feel that they can never stop doing. If they stop for even a moment, they fear that they will die or be left with nothing—which, to them, is as good as dying. The whole horror of existence can, for them, be summed up as failure. They will do anything to avoid failure, driven by what, to them, is no less than a survival instinct. They exist only because they do, and this is where their sense of worth resides. They fill their lives with stress and overload their schedules, making sure that they always have something to do, just so they won't feel a sense of emptiness.

Third-chakra types only know how to look at themselves from the outside. To a certain extent, they do not even have an "inside." Ironically, they are very proud of owning a strong sense of self—"I am an achiever; I am strong; I know what I want to do"—when they really don't have an inner self at all. They only have a social self—and, deep down, they know it. This terrifies them, and the only way to cope with the fear is to make sure they never have time to recognize it. They fill the empty gaps in their lives so they never have to face the fact that they can't exist without action and measurement. Because their biggest fear is emptiness, they simply fill their lives with even more activities and engage in even more competition.

The truth is that they just don't know any other way to live. They compensate for their fear with a sense of being successful—unlike all the "others." If they are not successful, they compensate with a confident assumption that they are near success. "Then" everyone else will be unimportant, while they will be a hero.

All the emotional traumas of the third type revolve around experiences of failure and powerlessness—moments and times when they were socially disrespected or even humiliated. To overcome this shadow self, they must first admit that they are empty inside and that they really don't know what to *do* with themselves.

They must start separating their sense of self from success and failure, and begin to form a self that is independent from all that. They also have to learn to accept failure, to honestly recognize that sometimes they *do* really fail and that they can be "losers" and still *be*.

Living eternally in the future, counting on becoming a great success "one day," is not a healthy way to live. The fact is that, even if third-chakra types are successful, they are still trapped in a state of inner hunger, since there is always someone above them on the social ladder, and there is no end to possibilities for growth and expansion. They must ask themselves what value there would be in life if they did, in fact, end up as failures. Failure and success depend on countless circumstances, and if you measure your life only against these values, you are already, in a way, a tragic failure.

The third type must learn to face emptiness. For this, they have to stop being proud of doing so much, having a packed schedule, and being importantly "busy." Their moment of truth comes when they realize that, by being busy, they simply run away from many real problems and neglect important areas in their lives.

Higher Potential and Destiny

Third-chakra types are here to teach everyone else how to believe in their own capacity for success. They guide us toward an optimal fulfillment of our inherent potential. In effect, they teach us the value and power of our own will.

To become a success, you must first acknowledge your will and then cultivate it as a unifying power that can focus all of your energies into one concerted effort. Achievers teach us to acknowledge our desires and show us that wanting is not a sin, but rather a crucial aspect of the manifestation of life and self. They teach us not only to acknowledge our desires, but to pursue them with all of our being. By daring to pursue our desires without compromise, we travel further on our journey of self-realization.

Achievers represent the divine aspect of victory, overcoming, empowerment, and evolution. They are able to awaken and inspire us to remember that we should never give up, despite all hindrances from within and without that seem to overpower our will. We need to acknowledge the spiritual value of victory, as well as embrace the process of overcoming obstacles as an inseparable part of the meaning of life. This includes not fearing the experience of failure, even if it hurts. They teach us always to aspire to the heights we are destined to reach and remind us how rewarding and elevating it can be when we are victorious. We tend to put the blame for our failures on circumstances. But Achievers tell us that the fulfilment of our hearts' wishes depends entirely on the qualities we bring to the journey.

They also provide us with the keys to shaping our own futures and to creating our fates, both as a race and as individuals. They tell us that we shouldn't blindly accept our so-called predetermined destiny, since so much of this destiny is in our own hands. From them, we learn that we hold the power to revolutionize patterns and pathways, and that "grace" does not lie only in the heavens, but also in humans taking full responsibility for their lives. Human evolution is grounded in people rising to new heights precisely because they recognize the need to go through a profound inner consolidation of themselves. And since grace manifests itself in human effort, those efforts are essentially beautiful and noble.

The third type shows us our self-dignity as it manifests in the capacity to overcome forces like laziness, fear, and stagnation. We achieve self-dignity by recognizing that we can always overcome weaknesses within ourselves and, by doing so, move to a new level through our own self-generated energy. By rising above the world of instincts, impulses, and desires, we do not "control," but rather transcend ourselves.

Achievers guide us to be courageous enough to become the heroes of our own stories by finding the hero within—the determined, fearless, immovable, and self-reliant self who is strong enough to move mountains.

Achieving Balance

There are several lifestyle changes that third-chakra types can make to balance the excesses in their constitution.

» Try to channel some of your energy of conquest inward. Learn to govern your instincts, impulses, fears, and anger. Strive for self-mastery, as opposed to constantly trying to be "number one" in the world.

» Find ways to transform your intense search for power into a quest for inner power. Learn who your real "enemies" are and where true "competition" takes place. Try to choose which battles you will fight and understand that the real victory in life is not achieved by conquering the outer world. External victories will never satisfy your deepest hunger, so avoid disillusionment and become a true hero by overcoming and conquering yourself.

» Avoid treating your inner forces and feelings with the same warrior-like approach with which you confront the outside world. A part of self-mastery is learning to let your energies flow, and harnessing them only when they become excessive or destructive.

» Learn to listen to your heart and cultivate the qualities of sensitivity, caring, and service. Adding emotions like love and selflessness to anything you do can transform the quality of your actions.

» Pay attention to partners, friends, children, and family or you may find yourself alone. The road to your goal is endless, so there is time for relationships even in the tightest schedule. Life is about more than just achieving and running forward.

» Avoid forcing your energy on others, whether that energy takes the shape of anger, rage, or even violence. Learn that what is good and right for you may not be good and right for anyone else. Finding an effective form of "anger management" can be crucial to your happiness.

» Look for other ways to direct your energies. Wisdom, meditation, vision, and love can reshape your raw powers. Great things can happen when your intensity is wisely harnessed and contained in some larger context.

» Remain humble and connect to some higher will in life. Because you are an active force that helps manifest abstract concepts in the world, you must use your energy to serve love and goodness so you can be of great help to all.

» Remember to keep the lighter parts of life active, including entertainment, laughter, and celebrations. Try to tap into the wisdom of the Artists. Don't skip vacations, and don't fall into the trap of "working vacations."

Finding Fulfillment

There are several paths that third-chakra types can follow to fulfill the potential of their constitution.

» Learn to relax—but not too much. Learn to lighten up without suppressing your natural and healthy high-voltage energy. You only need to curb your ambition and daring if you find yourself becoming self-destructive or egoistic. Otherwise, keep your fundamental intensity alive.

» Look for jobs that place you somewhere between the self-employed and being supervised. Try not to be completely constrained, so that you can feel as if you are pursuing your ambition. On the other hand, try to find a larger framework within which to work that can limit and guide your overflowing energy. As a visionary, you can become quite disoriented, so look for some worthy vision to carry out.

» When Achievers work as a team, they are like a pack of hungry wolves on the hunt. But you can channel this energy toward a good purpose by looking for challenges that are worth overcoming, goals that are worth achiev-ing, and honors that are worth garnering. What is import-ant is the possibility of achieving the unachievable and expanding without limits, barriers, or hindrances on the way. You live in the material world, not the mental world, so focus intently on making your goal a reality. You are practical and good at negotiating, so you can confidently translate any concept into an effective strategy for achiev-ing success.

» Your hyperactivity can sometimes be "too much" for others, so try to temper your tendency to become a workaholic, as this may negatively impact your relationships. If you give your partner a chance to appreciate your constitution, you'll experience greater harmony. Be willing to make a few sacrifices—especially time-related ones.

» Look for an ambitious spiritual path that is not purely passive and relaxing. Your spiritual pursuit should be an active process that combines striving with periods of relaxation, not just quiet contemplation or sinking into closed-eye meditation. Your instincts will be to follow a path that attempts to transform spiritual ideas into worldwide movements. Just make sure that goal doesn't overshadow your own actual practice. Your intense ambition can be a great advantage, so let it guide you. Just remember that spiritual attainment cannot be approached like other more earthly and materialistic goals.

» Learn to surrender your lower will and to sacrifice, to a certain extent, your proud individuality. Heart, wisdom, and consciousness are vital teachers as well, and can enable you to surrender your personal will to a higher cause and to sacrifice individuality when it becomes superfluous. Be cautious about your attraction to special powers and ways of subtle control through the spiritual path. Don't get stuck in miracle-working and other manipulations of reality. The true path is not about control over reality, but about becoming one with it.

» Strike a balance between your tendency to struggle with yourself and your need to accept and forgive yourself. The search for this balance may be the heart of your spiritual quest—taming the warrior cry you hear inside and accepting that which you cannot change.

Are You a Third-Chakra Personality?

This self-test will help you evaluate the percentage of the third-chakra type's presence in you. Let this moment of self-evaluation be relaxed and playful. Try not to evaluate the presence of this type in relation to other types. Just consider how much you recognize its characteristics in your way of being, your perception of the world, and your natural and immediate inclinations. Do not try to make an intellectual judgment. Trust that something in you will effortlessly recognize itself.

If you have trouble assigning a percentage to this chakra, read each of the following statements and questions and consider how closely you identify with them. If all your answers are 1s, you probably identify closely with the type. If all your answers are 4s, you probably don't. Use your responses to guide you in evaluating whether you belong to the third type. Once you have assigned a percentage, write it down so you can compare it with your other self-evaluations. This will help you determine your three-part personality type.

» I don't believe in good intentions; I want to see results. That is why marking a target and striving to conquer it with everything I've got is my experience of meaning in life.

1. Greatly identify

2. Moderately identify

3. Loosely identify

4. Cannot identify at all

» Are you constantly comparing yourself to others, examining who ranks below you and who ranks higher, while all the time wishing to become number one?

1. Definitely

2. Quite a bit

3. Perhaps a little

4. Not at all

» What would you say is the most active part in you?

1. Will and ambition

2. Mind and intellect

3. Body and feelings

4. Emotions

» Deep down, I am a warrior. My heroes are warriors and winners who fought uncompromisingly, even violently, for justice and freedom.

1. Definitely true

2. Quite true

3. Partially true

4. Not my experience at all

» When I enter a project, I can hardly breathe; I become an unstoppable fireball, impatient and pushy, and work at it tirelessly day and night. The sweat and effort exhilarate me!

1. Definitely

2. Yes, though I am conflicted about it

3. Perhaps true to a certain extent

4. Not at all

PART II

Emotional-Communicative Types

As we move from the world of the material-earthly types into the subtler world of the emotional-communicative types, we do not necessarily enter a "better" world. We just enter a world where a more refined type of interaction takes place. This middle group consists of the fourth and fifth chakra types—types who first encounter the world through emotions and fantasies. Both types' central passion in life is the act of communication. They strive to connect and bridge the inner and the outer worlds. Physically speaking, the emotional-communicative group corresponds to the chest, heart, lungs, and throat.

CHAPTER 4

FOURTH CHAKRA

The Caretakers

The Caretakers

» *Presence in world population:* around 15 percent

» *Public domain:* nonprofit organizations, charities and volunteer organizations, support groups, religious gatherings, therapy and healing

» *Typically found among:* therapists, healers, mediators, activists, volunteers, religious devotees, family people

» *Dosha constitution:* vata/kapha (air/water)

» *Dominated by:* the emotional center, heart

» *Shadow self:* the rejected giver

» *Time zone:* the present

» *Traditional animal:* antelope, deer

» *Famous figures:* Jesus, Jalal ad-Din Rumi, Teresa of Ávila, William Wilberforce, Yogananda, Florence Nightingale, Edith Cavell, David Livingstone, Mother Teresa, Padre Pio, Janusz Korczak, Etty Hillesum, Maximilian Kolbe, Dian Fossey, Patch Adams, Desmond Doss, Helen Keller, 14th Dalai Lama, Jane Goodall, Princess Diana, Mata Amritanandamayi, Thich Nhat Hanh

D espite belonging to the same group, the fourth and fifth chakra types are as different from each other as the first and second types are. Fifth-chakra types communicate because they want to influence, guide, and speak out. Fourth-chakra types communicate to realize their emotional potential. They don't care as much about influence as they do about intimacy.

Essence

The fourth chakra is located in the lower center of the chest and holds within it the essence of the unitive force. This force is easily seen in atoms, molecules, cells, and, more generally, in the biological world and animals. Its last and final expression is in the emotions. The unitive force is the binding force of the universe—the force of attraction that evokes an urge in different and separate elements to be pulled toward each other, to unify, and to become a greater whole.

At the atomic level, this force appears as electromagnetism, a strong force that binds atoms together. At the molecular level, it takes the form of the electrical and nuclear force. Behind all these physical forces is the binding force of the universe that works to connect energies, independent objects, and biological creatures. It is the force that allows them to cohere and develop new, increasingly whole, structures.

Our bodies, a creation of the unitive force, are truly a community of cells, which are communities of molecules, which are communities of atoms. These have all been drawn to participate in a certain project called "us." In the human world, this force drives people to form families, communities, nations, and other types of alliances. It is the force that encourages people to interact emotionally, intellectually, spiritually, and physically. This is also what Plato called the "madness of love." It is what makes us willing to lose our independence and autonomy, just so we can experience a precious oneness.

You feel this unitive urge as a need for emotional sharing—a readiness to leave behind your independence and freedom so you can feel that you are a part of something greater. This is the cause of our sometimes overwhelming passion for relationships and our need to communicate. Unlike the second-chakra essence, which similarly drives toward self-forgetfulness and loss of boundaries, this unitive force is a deeper longing for the act of sharing itself. We call it "intimacy"—the feeling that arises when we lose our sense of separation from one another.

Constitution

Fourth-chakra types are a mix of vata and kapha—air and water. On the one hand, they have a great deal of airiness that endows them with softness and roundedness, idealism and naiveté. On the other hand, they also have a wish for grounding. This type is not just about the lightness of emotions; they also experience a need to take root, to bring themselves into a definite expression.

Caretakers have a rounded appearance, with open and mellow features. Sometimes they have a tendency to fattiness. Their demeanor is relaxed and sweet, and their eyes are usually wide and soft. Being in their presence brings about a cooling and soothing energy, similar to that of a lake or a soft breeze. This inviting energy permeates you with the feeling that you can relax into it.

Sphere of Influence

Around 15 percent of the world's population is made up of fourth-chakra personalities. These people express and demonstrate the power of emotion and love. Their main passion is to bring people together, to unify, and to make sure that there is harmony all around.

Caretakers are commonly found among those who strive to form loving family units, raise children, cultivate friendships, and create opportunities for intimacy. They are extremely occupied with family interaction and the experience of committing to a partner in a romantic relationship.

A more intense expression of this personality is found among many activists, humanists, animal rights advocates, social dreamers, and world rectifiers—anyone who believes in world change and engages in the creation of movements for peace. Caretakers can never just sit quietly by and watch the world suffer. Their ideal is to "bring heaven to earth"; they believe that they can make this planet heavenly. Thus, all movements for world change have fourth-chakra types heavily involved. This is particularly true when this type is significantly influenced by the fifth type, whether as part of their personality blend or through external guidance. What propels these types as visionaries of world change, however, is much less some future utopian dream than identification with an emotional potential. They want to meet person-to-person; they want to come together and to feel and heal as one. What they are after is connection.

Caretakers are active in all fields of human connectivity and intimacy. They are therapists and healers, mediators and leaders of emotional group therapy. They are activists and volunteers, religious devotees and family people. Wherever you find them, however, they will most surely be immersed in some intense form of giving and devotion. Devotion is, in fact, their key experience, whether it be devotion to family, to children, to partners, or, more broadly, to people in need and to the world at large.

Another possible expression of this devotion is in certain spiritual and religious movements. Bhakti yoga (yoga of devotion) has made this drive toward devotion into a complete path to God through the cultivation of love and surrender to a guru, a deity, God, or humanity. Bhakti yoga was most definitely founded by fourth-chakra types who sought their own unique spiritual practice. Passionate about the gap between "me" and the "other"—the gap that gives rise to relationships—they explored the tension and union between "God" as the ultimate other and "me" as the devout believer. Followers of these types of religious movements are naturally the ultimate devotees.

In their most radiant form, Caretakers appear among those rare individuals who have given themselves heroically in expressions of self-sacrifice, universal compassion, and acts of faith. These paragons of selflessness have demonstrated an uncompromising willingness to sacrifice themselves, sometimes physically, for higher principles or for others in trouble. In doing so, they exhibit a great nobility of spirit.

Role in Human History

Historically, fourth-chakra types are highly active in developing the creator-soul relationship with a monotheistic God, including the sense of sin and virtue. Jesus, a key example of this type, transformed this relationship into one that is based in love, not law. In fact, in all religious and spiritual streams, Caretakers have brought forth their philosophies in practices like charity and service, prayers, devotional music, singing and chanting, and devotional poetry. Take, for example, the poetry of the Sufi master Jalal ad-Din Rumi.

Sufism in Islam, the Hassidic movement in Judaism, Mahayana Buddhism, and the Bahá'í Faith all put significant emphasis on the emotional center. The well-known "Bodhisattva Vow" in Mahayana Buddhism, in which an individual vows to incarnate endlessly until all sentient beings are released from the cycle of birth and death, is a striking expression of a fourth-type ideal.

During the 20th century, Caretakers have worked as active cocreators within different civil rights and peace movements, as well as in animal rights and ecological movements.

Worldview

Imagine the world as a space for emotional exchange—as if the whole world came into being just for sharing, just for giving and receiving. The driving force in such a world is relationships. Everything else is just a disturbance along the way. Of course, there are the realities of everyday living, but when it comes to *real life*, all that matters is what happens between "you" and "me," right now.

This is the world of the fourth personality type—a world where emotional experience is the heart of life and the center of human activity and communication. It is a world where the central happening is emotional exchange, even when it appears that people are meeting only for doing business. Beneath the superficial actions, it is all about that. Sometimes, loving your child or partner wholeheartedly and tending to their needs can be the most meaningful experience in your life. More often than not, this is where the truly powerful events of life await you, offering you a genuine path to development and transformation.

For Caretakers, love is the one true motivation in life. It is the search for love's fulfillment that drives them, for the simple reason that nothing else makes sense. Love is the first cause, the fuel, and the purpose. Therefore, there is absolutely no meaning in life as long as our hearts are empty. When we don't do everything we can possibly do to deepen our connection to others, we get stuck in a desolate desert, far away from the genuine purpose of life.

For a religious or spiritual fourth type, God, or spirit, is conceived of as love, and the ultimate achievement in life is to realize love in human form. This love is the only force that can overcome death, as it connects us to the stream of eternal love and an unbreakable soul connection. We can only contact this spirit through our hearts, and we can only be fulfilled through selfless love.

Caretakers find love—both religious and secular love—in feelings, as well as in actual devotion, caring, and service. They like to act in the name of devotion and to do things for others. They are not dreamy fifth-chakra types, however; they don't dwell in an abstract sense of love of God or humanity. For them, if love doesn't reach and flow into the material world, it is senseless. That is why their acts of love must be personal and individual. They need to bestow love and caring on an actual person or cause. Of course, that doesn't mean that they cannot be inspired by a universal vision of life. When Mother Teresa washed the lepers, she saw God in them. Although her devotion was universal, she didn't just sit and pray. She sought God in a human form in order to love and to serve. Likewise, even in charity work driven by a universal ideal, fourth-chakra types seek out individuals and strive to make them feel that they are personally significant.

Fourth-chakra types dwell in a unique position—at the midpoint between the universal and the personal. Put simply, their God has a face. For them, God is not the purely faceless spirit of the seventh-chakra type; nor is God the idealistic spirit of the fifth. Caretakers always exist in relationship; they need to relate. Even as religious devotees, they cannot abide an impersonal God. The divine, for them, must take a personal form. The spiritual experience of a fourth type is not found in the formless depths of meditation, but in a feeling of oneness with all and in an all-consuming love of God. Indeed, the mere yearning for unity fills them with the happy sense of connection to a greater whole.

Caretakers feel fulfilled only when they serve a cause greater than themselves, whether it is a family, a romantic relationship, humanity, or a deity. They always seek something of which they can become a part. Independence is an awkward concept to them, since they perceive life and the world as a web of interconnectedness. This also means that they find it hard to experience themselves as a "whole." In a way, a fourth-chakra type is like an incomplete being searching for its complementary half.

Naturally, Caretakers find life in a society like ours quite difficult and even hostile. Our society tends to disregard emotions and intimacy, and to prefer values like rationalism, achievement, individualism, self-satisfaction, and competitiveness. This can make fourth-chakra types feel quite alienated. In their hearts, they sense that this individuality has to melt into something greater or there can be no meaning to life. If an experience is not shared, if it remains isolated to one person, it has no meaning. Experience becomes real only when some other person hears about it or participates in it. And it becomes even more real when other people respond and share their sentiments about it. Then individuals can share this identical feeling, which brings about the happiest state in life—intimacy.

Moments of intimacy are not only the happiest times for fourth-chakra types. They are the only times when life becomes real. The ability to break through the barriers of separation, to look deeply into another's eyes and experience unity and a flood of emotional connectivity, is what Caretakers live for.

General Characteristics

We all know what it feels like to be a fourth-chakra type when we feel that being independent is not enough or that we cannot derive our true satisfaction from it. We recognize the type in ourselves when we feel a deeper sense of satisfaction and need to share it and perhaps even to experience it with another person, even at the price of losing our sense of power, sovereignty, and independence. Whenever the binding force manifests in us and drives us to seek intimacy—with lovers, friends, family, children, group, or community—we become fourth-chakra types. We meet this type in ourselves when we yearn for world peace or dream of how people can live together without separation to create a global community. We find the unitive force within when we attempt to gather the many human atoms into one molecule of humanity.

Because Caretakers are dominated by their emotional center, their sense of existence can be defined as, "I feel strongly toward someone, therefore I am." These personalities exist in relation, through their connection to the "other." They need others out there to love, to think about, to go to for recognition. They love this interplay of duality, even while they seek to experience final unity with their beloved.

Fourth-chakra types are highly sensitive beings, and when their emotional center overflows, they can become overly sensitive. They always feel something and can't understand people who don't feel sometimes. This can bring conflict into their relationships, because they simply cannot comprehend it when someone lacks feeling at a certain moment. This prompts in them a burning desire to fix what they sense is broken in the other person. Caretakers have to learn to accept that others are not meant to share their worldview, especially since, even when others around them evince feelings, they are never as intense as their own.

The fourth-chakra type's capacity for intimacy is far greater than that of most other types, with the exception, perhaps, of Artists. They are friendly and warm, simple-hearted, interested, and chatty. Inevitably, their conversations tend to put their emotions and feelings about things at the center—along with those of others—as this is the only way they understand intimacy. In sexuality, they find it hard to separate the sexual act from the emotional encounter and so require deep familiarity and trust to engage in sex comfortably.

In general, Caretakers communicate with the world around them through intense emotions, and this is also the way they evaluate truth and falsity. If they feel strongly about something, it must be true, and this evaluation influences the way they make decisions and choices. Even when they try to go through a long and thoughtful process of consideration, it is their feelings that carry the day. At their best, they are good father and mother figures who bestow caring and support on others. They are gifted with a high sensitivity to the suffering of others and are capable of beautiful expressions of compassion. They are attracted to volunteer work and most probably were the first ones to raise their hands at school when some task was offered.

Like Builders, Caretakers tend to be practical and to give a lot of attention to the small details of life, although they do this not to achieve an undisturbed balance, but rather out of a natural instinct to be of service. Another similarity between Builders and Caretakers is their fondness for rituals and ceremonies, and their "tribal consciousness." They value belonging to a greater family, whether a biological family or a group of soul mates and friends.

Strengths and Gifts

The fourth type radiates sweetness, and others usually find their presence cooling and relaxing. They are naturally attentive and considerate, so it is always nice to be pampered by them. Those chosen by them as their dearest will surely benefit from their devotional spirit and the many selfless acts and gestures made toward them. They are gentle, peaceful, and harmonious. They find quarrels and tensions intolerable and will do anything in their power to put an end to them. While other, prouder, types may insist that they are right in almost every argument, fourth-chakra types don't much care who is right. They are far more concerned with maintaining a lasting state of peace in which no one is ever angry.

Caretakers are also innocent almost to the point of being naive. They generally believe in the inherent goodness of others and seek their deeper motives when they do wrong. They approach situations in life with an optimistic spirit, tending to feel that everything will eventually work out for the best.

Challenges

When their emotional centers overflow, fourth-chakra types can quite easily become overly emotional and hover on the verge of hysteria. In this state of hypersensitivity, their every emotion risks becoming disproportionate. As much as they feel love, this type also feels excruciating and tearful pain. To less emotional types, this can surely be seen as excessive, which merely annoys them and makes them even more emotionally disturbed.

In relationships, Caretakers are very devoted. On the other hand, they can be extremely demanding. Less emotional types who engage in relationships with them often feel as if they are always expected to engage in some sort of exchange. At moments like these, when the emotional thread seems to be "broken," fourth-chakra types tend to drift into a distorted and dramatic interpretation of the situation, feeling that everything is destroyed or that something is terribly wrong in the world.

Caretakers can also be intensely jealous and possessive toward their chosen ones—and even somewhat violent if they feel in danger of losing them. They are caught in a vicious circle. They are by nature sensitive and vulnerable, and as a result, they can feel dependent and helpless. They try to compensate for this by making childish demands and by using blame and anger as a form of "violence of the weak." This dependency and helplessness can also lead them to be passive followers of others with a more determined will, which leads to another vicious circle, as it inevitably brings about feelings of anger and rebellion.

Fourth-chakra types have difficulty thinking logically, because they are guided by the heart and the emotional center. This makes them quite irrational and unable to detach from blinding emotions. They can indulge in the world of emotions so much that they eventually become utterly absorbed in their internal experience—what they feel about another and how things make them feel—while, ironically, remaining completely oblivious to the other person's state. When this happens, they forget that emotions are there to connect people and not to enhance self-obsession and separation from others. When their gift of sensitivity and compassion is no longer turned toward others, but rather toward themselves, they can be filled with self-pity and an acute neediness.

The fourth type can be obsessive in relationships. This is reflected in their mental activity, which tends to become immersed in overthinking relationships. If you could see inside their daily thought patterns, you would probably find that they think mostly about other people and the status of their relationships with them. If you point this out to them, they will probably be surprised: "What else could I think about? Isn't that what all people think about?"

Sometimes their naiveté can be excessive. Their fervent belief in the goodness of others—that others couldn't possibly mean to do wrong—can lead them to make wrong judgments. For them, it can be a tough and painful lesson from life that, at this stage of mankind's development, some people do actually intend to do bad things. Since, in general, they are somewhat like naive children who expect and want to believe that everything is rosy, they are easily led into blind optimism when making choices in life.

Shadow Self

Caretakers always need to love and be loved. In fact, they spend their entire lives seeking confirmation of the fact that they are truly loved. And their greatest fear is that they will be rejected. That is why I call their shadow self "the rejected giver."

To avoid rejection, Caretakers simply give, give, give all the time. This is what motivates their sacrifice and their focus on others. It may seem that they are "all about others," but there is, in fact, a hole in their hearts that derives from tremendous insecurity. This hole keeps them continually off-balance and unsure, and that is why they always feel guilty that they are not giving enough. If they only gave enough, they reason, they would be loved enough.

This insecurity is grounded in the fact that they are not sure who they are without interaction with another. Take away all others and they panic: "Who am I? What is happening to me? I am dissolving!" This inevitably leads to a state of constant insecurity, which then compels them to search for a final confirmation that they are loved. The problem is that even God cannot grant them confirmation that will satisfy them, because their insecurity is actually a part of their nature. Even if God descended from the heavens to reassure them, this would not bring them a sense of security or a release from the need for further confirmation. This was the case with Mother Teresa, whose life of sacrifice was at least partly driven by the insecurity of not being loved by God. Her letters reveal a disturbing feeling of being rejected by God, and this insecurity transformed into a compulsion to give. This is often the case with our gifts—they are inextricably linked to our psychological needs.

Fourth-chakra types compensate for their insecurity by making themselves into martyrs. They are, of course, very proud of being givers, selflessly giving everything away. This sort of giving is valued by society. But what seems on the surface to be a pure and noble love, love for the sake of love, is really a need to be loved themselves, motivated by a fear of rejection.

The most unbearable experience for this chakra type is to be unloved and rejected. When they are rejected, they feel as if they are as good as dead. The main psychological work for this type is to admit their insecurity and recognize that their love and their giving are not purely noble. They need to acknowledge that they are often motivated by dependency, insecurity, and addiction. They must also learn to accept the feeling of rejection and know that, even when someone appears to reject them, they still remain alive and breathing.

It is unwise to live in a state in which you depend on another for confirmation of your own existence. That is why Caretakers need to cultivate a sense of self that exists without others. Although it is not in their nature to be fully independent, they need to strive for some level of self-existence. Finally, they must recognize that they are not going to receive any final confirmation of the fact they are loved. This is a need that simply cannot be met. Once they realize this, they can work to purify their beautiful instinct to give.

Higher Potential and Destiny

Fourth-chakra types are our greatest teachers when it comes to the fullness of the heart. Blessed with the intuition that, without an overflowing heart, nothing makes sense, they help us to complete our picture of the meaning of life. They teach us that devotion is the key to filling our hearts with meaning. Without devotion—without the urge to devote ourselves to something larger than ourselves and to serve it—we can never overcome the disturbing sense of emptiness and isolation in our hearts. They also teach us that, as long as we do not open ourselves to love, we miss out, not only on an essential component of genuine self-fulfillment, but also on our connection to a meaningful life.

This chakra type emerged from the cosmic dimension of unity—the love that melts away boundaries and can overcome the forces of separation, alienation, and loneliness in the world. They are the world's unifiers, whose role is to make us transcend petty differences and realize that our common ground is far greater than our individual existences.

This common ground of unity can only be revealed when we agree to allow an emotional sharing, when we allow ourselves to engage in an intimate, exposed, sensitive, and attentive exchange. Merely exchanging information, thoughts, and opinions only widens the gap between us, however. It is emotional sharing that helps remove our social masks and shows that, behind them, we are essentially the same. Other types don't know how to do this very well, but the Caretakers endow us with an awareness of emotional intelligence. They help us master the many intricacies and subtleties of interpersonal relationships and achieve openness and mutual understanding.

The fourth type encourages us to be more accepting toward people as they are, at whatever point they are, and helps us see the deeper nature and goodness in them beyond superficial appearances. By bringing the healing power of acceptance to our world, they help us heal the wounds of brutal competition, comparison, and inferiority. They bring us the gift of forgiveness and show us how we can overcome our righteous opinions and prefer the sweetness and softness of unification, even with those who appear to be our enemies.

Caretakers evoke in us the inner call for activism—for actual action in the face of suffering—and remind us that we cannot sit idly by and watch a world in pain. Dreaming of world peace accomplishes nothing; world peace begins in our smallest actions of kindness. They call us to be attentive to the suffering of others, to remove the wall that stands between our hearts and the world and keeps us apathetic and self-immersed. They make us notice what is happening around us.

Caretakers show us love as a boundless source of energy and power. Too often, we act from motivations like ambition and desire. Yet love, they tell us, can move mountains. When we act out of love, there is no sense of effort. Seen from their perspective, caring only for our own interests causes us to disengage from a source of endless life-force that only those who dedicate their lives to others can know. When we tap into this source and serve wholeheartedly, we realize that whatever energy we give flows back to us. This love is not something we need to receive, but rather an abundant force within us. It is always our choice whether to tap into it or not.

The fourth chakra gives us the gift of conscience, with its added values of friendship, faithfulness, nonviolence, and sacrifice. It reminds us of the beauty of commitment—what it means to devote our lives to others until we breathe our last. It also bestows on us the gift of the soul, reminding us all of our relationship with a higher reality, a relationship we fulfill through prayer, faith, and service. It whispers in our ears the secret teaching that, as souls, we can achieve self-fulfillment only when we devote our lives to something greater than ourselves.

Fourth-chakra personalities show us a vision of a planet based on love, and a human culture driven by the law of love. Even if you don't belong to this type and may never become an endless giver, they can inspire you to start with some small acts of kindness. Even if we cannot completely dedicate our lives to something greater than ourselves as ideal examples of the fourth type do, they inspire us to have at least some larger meaning and deeper service in one area of our lives. And even if we cannot see the oneness in everyone and forgive all who do us wrong, as they do (often in astonishing ways), they guide us to forgive—at least sometimes.

Achieving Balance

There are several lifestyle changes that fourth-chakra types can make to balance the excesses in their constitution.

» The most important balancing work for you as a Caretaker is to balance your emotional excess. First, learn to direct your natural-born sensitivity. Try not to turn inward in an unhealthy way. Remember that this is really a gift that is meant to be directed toward others in the form of compassion and attentiveness to their suffering.

» Don't assume that your energy flows naturally toward others. Being obsessed with a relationship and wanting to know that someone loves you has nothing to do with caring for someone. Remember to embrace this universal law: whenever you want to feel love, don't ask for love; just love.

» Make sure your sensitivity takes the form of some sort of activism—anything you feel is a noble cause, any purpose greater than yourself. Join a world movement that strives for change, or pursue some smaller activities that encourage an emotional flow toward others to prevent stagnation. Learn to associate your truest source of happiness with altruistic activities.

» Understand that love is action and not a mere feeling, as powerful as that feeling may be. Don't content yourself with entering the world of feelings; you must take the next step and translate those feelings into action. To help channel your emotional energy, ask yourself the question: "What can I do?"

» Learn to minimize excessive indulgence in personal relationships, although this may not be easy for you. Don't become overly invested in your relationships and neglect to cultivate your independence. Don't expend all your energy on intense interpersonal engagements and exchanges. Sometimes you have to give some space, both to yourself and to others.

» Don't put your need for emotional fulfillment on one poor man or woman, since no one can possibly take on the burden of such unrealistic expectations. And be careful not to force your own expectations for emotional exchange on others. Not everyone shares your intense sentiments. Trying to "convert" a partner who is not as emotional as you are into a fervent believer in emotions is just not fair.

» If your emotions overflow, try attending a seminar that offers practices of intimacy and loving exchange. Join a community or even turn to a passionate pet like a dog who will always share your feelings. Accept yourself and understand that, as a fourth-chakra personality, you experience a great need and hunger for emotional exchange. But don't try to fill that need with only one person. It must be spread around.

» Your type is prone to severe feelings of being unwanted, separate, and deserted, but you must resist the expectation that your soul mate can fill this hole in your heart. This can lead to frustration and, ironically, to a breakup. Only a few can stand up to the expectation that they are, in fact, the only important person in the world and the sole support of someone else's sense of existence.

» Look for relationships with both the inner and outer spirit and widen your horizons as much as possible. An active spiritual connection with a higher force—prayer, meditation, chanting—can also answer your deeper need for final unity and wholeness on the soul level. Because you inherently experience yourself as an incomplete being, reach out to spirit to find your other half.

» Learn to let go. Your unbalanced tendency is to cling to things too strongly and to fix your attention permanently on the one who loves you. This makes for strong commitment and loyalty, but maintaining a fixation on past lovers and other connections can be damaging as well. Learn to walk away from damaging relationships and to recognize, not only the beauty of faithfulness, but also its inherent fear of being without your other half. When something ends, dare to leave it behind and remember that true love can never be a fixation.

» Resist the temptation to sacrifice yourself for another or for a cause. The tendency to give yourself away is beautiful, but it is not always heroic to "kill" yourself. Heroic stories of martyrs may seem ennobling. But remember that, too often, you become a martyr for far less good reason.

» Above all, learn to love yourself. While it is clearly harmful to overindulge in your inner emotional world, it is still vital that you direct love and acceptance toward yourself. When you turn your love and acceptance only to others, forgetting yourself, you misunderstand the true meaning of caring.

» Try not to be too naive. Accept that, from time to time, people can be bad. You may argue that it's not people who are bad, only their actions, but at least remember to be realistic about your own relationships.

» Accept that you don't really need to exist in an uninter-rupted state of peace, love, and harmony. Sometimes friction, whether in a relationship or in a developmental process, is necessary to attain greater love and harmony.

» Avoid building a protective wall around your heart to deal with your many strong emotions and disappointments. Learn that being vulnerable and open can be more pro-tective than any wall. Let go of your defenses and try to remain vulnerable. Keep your heart open and love even when it doesn't make sense.

» Seek out trustworthy mentors to help you mature the more childish elements of your emotional center. Mentoring can keep you focused as you transition from being the one in need to being the one who gives to others.

Finding Fulfillment

There are several paths fourth-chakra types can follow to fulfill the potential of their constitution.

» If you are aware that you are not good at handling business on your own, seek help from a capable first-chakra type. Don't push yourself into trying to be something you can never be. To a reasonable extent, follow your intuition that life is less about money and much more about doing something you believe in.

» Seek success in professions that channel the emotions and lead to sharing—healers, caretakers, and therapists of all kinds. Consider a career in medicine. Follow your inclination to guide people through emotional therapy or intimacy and accompany them on their journeys of recovery or even of dying. You will be successful working with children (including in education), as a social activist, working with animals, and in family and couples therapy.

» Avoid relationships that suppress your nature. Getting stuck in a highly unemotional connection, or even an abusive and violent one, can steadily drain your life-force.

» In business and in relationships, follow your basic nature, which encourages you to collaborate with others. Though you clearly need to liberate yourself from stifling dependency, at the same time you must honor the fact that the growth in your life takes place through some other or others.

» Try a spiritual path like Bhakti yoga—the path of love, surrender, and devotion. Identify some object of devotion—a teacher, a deity, or even humanity. Incorporate chanting and other types of devotional music into your practice and seek emotional unity with others. Perform your meditations with your eyes open to maintain your tie to the real world.

» Avoid spiritual paths that are purely emotional, with no systematic or clear wisdom, as they may leave you helpless and not knowing how to interpret your experience. Make sure that your path involves some form of active service so you don't get stuck in feelings with no way to channel them. Look for perfect models of self-sacrifice to illuminate your unique path of the heart.

Are You a Fourth-Chakra Personality?

This self-test will help you evaluate the percentage of the fourth-chakra type's presence in you. Let this moment of self-evaluation be relaxed and playful. Try not to evaluate the presence of this type in relation to other types. Just consider how much you recognize fourth-chakra characteristics in your way of being, your perception of the world, and your natural and immediate inclinations. Do not try to make an intellectual judgment. Trust that something in you will effortlessly recognize itself.

If you have trouble assigning a percentage to this chakra, read each of the following statements and questions and consider how closely you identify with them. If all your answers are 1s, you probably identify closely with the type. If all your answers are 4s, you probably don't. Use your responses to guide you in evaluating whether you belong to this personality type. Once you have assigned a percentage, write it down so you can compare it with your other self-evaluations. This will help you determine your three-part personality type.

» The world is a space of emotional bonding, and we are here to realize our maximum potential as love in a human form.

   1. Greatly identify

   2. Moderately identify

   3. Loosely identify

   4. Cannot identify at all

» What would you say is the most active part in you?

   1. Emotions

   2. Feelings and body

   3. Will and ambition

   4. Mind and intellect

» My ideal way of sharing my being with others is . . .

   1. A one-on-one personal and intimate engagement in which we open our hearts to one another

2. A circle of people who discuss or create together with an empathic spirit and a sense of shared vision

3. Teaching others face-to-face, while also being emotionally open

4. Engaging in a profound philosophical discussion with a thoughtful person

» I am most happy when I manage to make others happy.

1. Exactly my experience

2. Quite true

3. Somewhat true

4. Not my experience at all

» I feel that my process of development happens through some other or others—a soul mate, a friend, or a teacher; this is my path to growth.

1. Perfectly true

2. Quite true

3. Only to some degree

4. Not at all

CHAPTER 5

FIFTH CHAKRA

The Speakers

The Speakers

» *Presence in world population:* around 7 percent

» *Public domain:* media, education, politics, social media, court

» *Typically found among:* journalists, authors, teachers, principals, politicians, judges, lawyers, salesmen, singers

» *Dosha constitution:* vata/pitta (air/fire)

» *Dominated by:* the communicating center, voice

» *Shadow self:* the all-controlling manipulator

» *Time zone:* the distant future

» *Traditional animal:* singing birds, wolf

» *Famous figures:* the biblical Isaiah, John the Baptist, Solon, Mohamed, Niccolo Machiavelli, William Shakespeare, Henry David Thoreau, Martin Luther, Karl Marx, Fyodor Dostoyevsky, Beethoven, Gabriel García Márquez, Mahatma Gandhi, Osho, Martin Luther King Jr., Malcolm X, John F. Kennedy, John Lennon, Nelson Mandela, Carl Sagan, Steve Jobs, Bill Gates, Mark Zuckerberg, Deepak Chopra, Tony Morrison, Oprah Winfrey, Barack Obama, Elon Musk, Barbara Marx Hubbard, Ray Kurzweil

Speakers share an essential similarity with Caretakers. Their central passion in life is the act of communication. However, the two types approach communication in very different ways. Whereas fourth-chakra personalities find communication fulfilling only when it becomes an opportunity for emotional intimacy, fifth-chakra personalities experience fulfillment when they get the chance to influence people and events. For them, meetings with others are opportunities to make themselves heard, in the hope that they can change their listeners' minds or touch their hearts. They cherish communication less than its effects—its degree of influence and the success of the idea or vision they are voicing. Another way to say it is that, while Caretakers communicate in order to connect with others, Speakers communicate in order to give full expression to their own thoughts and feelings.

Essence

The fifth chakra lies at the base of the throat. It is here that we find an essential element of existence with which we are constantly in touch, yet tend to take for granted—*language*.

Think for a moment how much we express ourselves through language. Every thought, idea, and feeling we experience is voiced in words, whether we use those words to explain our own elusive feelings to ourselves or to explain ourselves to others. Language connects our inner world with another's inner world. It is the glue that binds together different realities by creating a bridge of understanding.

The fifth-chakra essence is more than the language of words, however. It is any form of exchange of information—all those shared codes that all forms of life use to communicate. Mushrooms and trees in the forest share information. Birds constantly send signals to each other. Through voices, gestures, and even sub-tle energies, all conscious beings speak to one another. Indeed, human language has become so complex that it can share not only information about survival and function, but also abstract ideas and values.

At this very moment, as you are reading these lines, we are both activating our fifth-chakra essence. I am using carefully selected words to fulfill my declared intention to affect your con-sciousness, and shape and direct it. It is nothing short of magic that we can change each other's minds through a set of letters and sounds. Every word I utter creates a reality in you. What we express through language can change that reality.

Language is so powerful that it can gather people into world-wide organizations, make them form unions, and encourage them to join movements. To activate this magic, of course, you must use the right language—the exact words that will touch everyone at the same time and in the same way. But even this is not enough. To convince different people from different worlds to gather and act in concert requires a secret ingredient called "charisma"—the power to enchant your listeners with your presence as well as your words. Through charismatic speech, you can evoke feelings that are exactly what people want to feel, even if they don't know they want to feel it. Naturally, whoever wields this charismatic power controls the transmission of ideas and information within the cul-ture and can therefore direct it at will.

Everyone tries to influence the people and events around them, whether consciously or unconsciously, when they express opinions or feel urged to share their inner beliefs, ideals, or vision. This is the essence of the fifth personality—a burning passion to affect the world around them.

Constitution

The constitution of the fifth-chakra personality is a combination of vata and pitta (air and fire). They possess a great deal of the fire element, which manifests itself in their wish to express ideas, and influence and inflame others. At the same time, they are also very airy, far from grounded, and reluctant to plant their ideas in the earthly soil.

Physically speaking, fifth-chakra types are strong, solid, straightforward, and wakeful. Their facial outlines are usually sharp and they have a sharp look as well. They tend to be very outward-looking, as if they stand with their faces turned to the world. They possess a high awareness of their surroundings and of the many things that happen around them. They are sensitive to other people's responses as well because of their constant need to "work" with their feedback.

Speakers tend to be thin, although they can have a tendency to overweight. And they are always energetic. When entering a room, they are a bit like politicians who come ready to shake hands. They have a certain diplomatic demeanor, since, in many respects, they feel that they are forever in need of impressing others and bringing about fruitful outcomes through communication. Full of intention, they never just speak to you; they always want something and always have a "plan." Even when they pretend that their interactions are purely social—and they are efficient pretenders—they always want to influence outcomes and achieve certain goals.

In this, they are the opposites of Artists, who never really care about outcomes and just want to have fun. When a Speaker speaks to you, prepare to be manipulated. Here, they far exceed the Achievers, who are not necessarily such good communicators and are relatively transparent. You can recognize a fifth-chakra type by the way they approach you with the clear intention of making you feel as if they are *really* interested in speaking to you and listening to you.

Sphere of Influence

Speakers constitute only around 7 percent of the world's population. Due to their leading roles and media presence, however, they seem to be everywhere. They make ideas run through a culture, functioning as bridges between concepts and people.

In his 1976 book *The Selfish Gene*, evolutionary biologist Richard Dawkins, himself a clear fifth personality type, coined the term "meme" to capture the self-replicating, gene-like nature of ideas. He argued that ideas spread from person to person within a culture in a way similar to biological evolution. Just like other living organisms like viruses, they seek hosts—in this case, our brains—and have an instinct for self-preservation.

Memes are successful when someone manages to implant an idea in people's minds in such a way that it takes hold of them and uses them as carriers to pass the idea on until it secures its roots within the culture. Speakers are good at meme creation and are behind the spread of many of them. Even Dawkins's meme, which is an idea about ideas, has managed to take root. In fact, I am demonstrating the process by passing it on to you right now!

All good lecturers and leaders have fifth-chakra characteristics, whether as their major or their secondary personality type. A proficient lecturer or leader must be able to make many people follow one ideal, even if that ideal is really self-interest disguised as an idea (a symptom of a likely fifth-type imbalance). All fifth-chakra types are potential leaders, although, of course, that doesn't mean that every member of this type will grow into a magnetic and charismatic leader. Yet, they all share some level of this magnetic power—the capacity to find the right words by perceiving the needs of those right in front of them.

This capacity makes them highly manipulative. When you know exactly what someone needs and wants to hear, you can easily use that knowledge to tempt and convince. Where this skill is used for good purposes and idealistic causes, we find great leaders who speak in the name of truth and often bring about positive world change. At the same time, we can find this very same capacity to direct and inspire in those who abuse it by implanting ideas that are dangerous or destructive.

The controversial 20th-century spiritual teacher Osho was a fifth-chakra type who demonstrated these two extremes. Probably the greatest manipulator of all spiritual teachers in history, he gave eloquent speeches in which he contradicted himself over and over, making outrageous statements that he then dismissed altogether. A professional debater in his early years, he traveled throughout India just to partake in religious debates, believing far less in the accuracy of his statements than in their power to affect people's minds. His whole way of speaking—from his hypnotic voice to his soothing hand gestures—was unashamedly manipulative.

Fifth-chakra types are also found among influential artists, in particular those who use art to express their opinions and oppose social and political injustice. John Lennon's eternal song *Imagine* is an example of such a statement taking the form of art. Lennon, unquestionably a fifth type, was much more than a great musician. He wasn't content with writing and singing about romantic heartbreak. He was a representative of an entire generation who gave voice to a more general revolution. Another excellent example is Toni Morrison, who is not only a gifted novelist, but also one who uses her voice to speak out for oppressed black people and relate their tragic history.

Second-chakra types are often artists for the pure sake of art as an unrestrained creative eruption, as in the case of comedian Andy Kaufman or musician Jim Morrison. By contrast, when fifth-chakra types express themselves through art, they tend to sustain that creative energy and apply it to far more complex works. They also know how to harness and channel it in order to make a clear statement. They have agendas to which they may dedicate their whole lives. Indeed, they may only write, sing, or compose because they want to make a point.

Speakers are often effective "translators" and explainers of systems. A part of their beauty is that they know exactly how to translate ideas and methods into a common language that many can grasp. They can pick up a certain complex notion—from science or mysticism, for example—and quickly translate it into a meme that will capture the minds and imaginations of many. When they stumble across a good concept, they immediately ask themselves how people might learn it and be influenced by it.

Not only are they superb explainers and interpreters of systems, but they also know how to connect one idea to another to form a synthesis. They like blending methods, systems, and ideologies to create new hybrid ideas. This is their unique form of innovation. They are able to bring together different methods—even some that seem diametrically opposed to one another. They learn a concept from one system and "translate" it in their minds into the language of another system—for instance, explaining a scientific principle in terms that spiritual people can understand, or spiritual concepts in a way that scientists can appreciate. Deepak Chopra gives a good example of this in his integration of ancient yogic principles into a scientific framework, blending elements of Western and Eastern thought.

Many fifth-chakra types become representatives of and speakers for systems. While sixth-chakra types (Thinkers) prefer to do their innovative thinking in the background, Speakers always want to put themselves forward. As manifestors, they are keenly interested in visibility. Most books have been written by Speakers rather than Thinkers. While Thinkers create ideas, Speakers explain them.

Speakers are found in abundance among teachers, guides, coaches, experts, and educators of all sorts. They love to teach—whether children or adults—and they take a particular interest in children because they are easy to shape. They are also copywriters, publicists, critics, journalists, publishers, and translators. Their fondness for "putting on a show" may also lead them to become stage performers, salespeople, judges, and lawyers (specifically those who like to perform in court).

Fifth-chakra types often serve as the voice of a "higher source." They may be prophets, channelers, and visionaries. In general, they like speaking "in the name" of something greater than themselves or for some clear good. Since defending a greater truth is a passion for them, they are often found speaking out against social and political injustice, vehemently representing values of freedom and human or animal rights. Contemporary animal rights activist Gary Yourofsky is known to be such an influential proponent of veganism that many people who watch his lectures online are "converted" by him. As visionaries, fifth-chakra types can be highly inspiring and can give direction to humanity as a whole, pointing out how far we can go and marking out new horizons.

This very tendency also leads them to become missionaries, feeling they are the saviors of mankind. They often preach some form of salvation—Christian, Jewish, or Muslim. What motivates them, however, is not the saving of souls, but the challenge of spreading their meme. They like to chart the growing number of believers in their cause, as they naturally think in terms of global changes. When this missionary spirit is expressed through great men like Martin Luther King Jr. or Gandhi, who also had a tremendous heart, the results can be remarkable. When it is expressed by sleazy politicians or "divinely inspired" inquisitors, the results are less uplifting.

Role in Human History

Speakers revealed their unique skills as soon as humanity started to expand its use of language beyond survival needs and began to create tribal hierarchies. At that point, they emerged to influence collective decisions and values, splitting into two major camps—leaders and their opposition. We can see this clearly in the Bible, where prophets arose to confront kings and religious leaders.

In ancient Greece, the delivery of speeches became a significant cultural event, with orators gathering in the Agora to draw people together and provoke discussion. The early elements of democracy appeared as citizens began to partake in the process of decision-making and to give voice to the worldview of the common people. Later, conventional fifth-chakra leaders who spoke for the established hierarchy diverged from unconventional fifth-chakra types who fought for social justice in important times of transition like the French Revolution and the American Civil Rights Movement. Today, we are immersed in fifth-chakra rhetoric because of an explosion in individual expression enabled by social media and supported by a widespread notion of self-fulfillment.

Worldview

Imagine the world as a space defined by opportunities for expression. In this space, many unique voices struggle to be heard, recognized, and accepted. Sometimes these individual voices even try to suppress each other. Each voice wants to be heard—to stand out—and to use its unique expression to influence people and events, and make changes in reality and in the way others think and behave.

It is this possibility of making a change that drives fifth-chakra types. They each have a unique inner vision that has the potential to affect both their lives and those of others. One may be a dreamer who sees the possibility of a new or enhanced reality. Another may be convinced that, if only everyone would adopt his vision, the world would be a different and better place. Whatever their vision, Speakers are all driven to promote it in order to make a change in the world. For them, it is all about following their own voice and inner vision and persuading others to follow it as well. They each "sing their own song"—sometimes loud and clear—but they also want others to sing along with them.

For fifth-chakra types, the dream must be followed at all costs—sometimes even after death. Their dreams, when focused on a great enough goal, are a legacy that continues after they are gone because it has meaning for others. These dreams are rooted so deeply in the far-off future that they can never be fully attained in one lifetime, but they remain behind as a hope that the Speaker's unique voice and message will be remembered and cherished.

Fifth-chakra types who are spiritual or religious connect with a higher reality by finding their own deepest and most personal expression. By doing so, they believe that they recognize the imprint of the divine in themselves—the uniqueness of their souls as an expression of God's true will. For them, to love is to allow others to sing their own song, too and to totally express their innermost selves. To follow the divine, you must give voice to truth, not just experience it yourself. If you are able to perceive something that seems like truth, you must spread the word. Their driving passion is to avoid keeping their own inner truth trapped inside themselves, and to share it with as many others as possible, as convincingly as possible.

Speakers find happiness in those moments in life that provide an opportunity to give voice to a natural flow of expression—something that makes others respond deeply. For them, this is almost like the experience of giving birth. In a sense, when others recognize and accept their inner truth, knowledge, and wisdom, they are inseminated by it and bring forth fruitful change.

Speakers also find happiness when they succeed in gathering a group of unique individuals and connecting them by making them understand and appreciate each other. For them, creating these bridges is the ultimate form of service. Touching someone else's mind and heart is a reflection of their ability to be a good channel for ideas. This is a major path to self-fulfillment for this personality type—being a channel for some idea or truth and letting it flow undisturbed.

Speakers envision the world as a space for manifestation. Beyond the act of giving expression to a certain idea or dream, they hope that their visions will take root in the world. That is why they seek to "organize" their beliefs, forming structures and movements that can deepen their impact on others and on the world. Their dreams start as seeds within their minds and then seek expression. If they are successful, those dreams will finally manifest in the world. Like the biblical God who gave rise to creation through the *logos*, or word, they seek to change reality through the expression of their thoughts. For God, however, there was no gap between expression and manifestation. For Speakers, who live in a world of matter resistant to change, the process is often a slow and painful one.

General Characteristics

We were all fifth-chakra types during our childhood, adolescence, and early twenties, when we harbored big dreams about how far we would go in our lifetimes. We wanted to conquer the world and felt that the sky was the limit. As we grow older, however, we tend to grow more cynical in response to life's increasing demands and the painful compromises we have to make along our paths of self-fulfillment.

We are all fifth-chakra types as well when we find ourselves searching for "our own voice" and unique expression. This begins in adolescence and young adulthood, when we look for our own meaning and fulfillment, our passions and abilities, through the choices we make regarding studies and work. We and others around us sense a "potential" in us that awaits exploration. And there are certain times of crisis in our lives when we realize that our potential has been buried beneath duties and expectations. So we sometimes find ourselves striving once again to "come out" into the world.

We are all fifth-chakra types when we are excited to learn that things we did or said have managed to guide or make a change in someone else's life. We are fifth personalities when we succeed in giving a clear form to some inner truth that is very dear to us and feel the joy of self-realization, or when we achieve the visible manifestation of a creative project and receive external confirmation that we have managed to reach others' hearts and minds. We also find the fifth type in ourselves when we have a grand vision for the future of the world and humanity, and are thrilled at the prospect of bringing about a more utopian reality.

An easy way to visualize the character of the fifth-chakra type is through the image of a battlefield. There is a commander who sits in a tent with maps spread before him, studying the situation and guiding his officers. But there is also an active field commander who goes into battle with his soldiers. The field commander is a third-chakra type, while the strategist is a fifth-chakra type who subtly guides from behind the scenes. While the third type is a highly energetic and fearless soldier who bravely rushes toward death, the fifth type is far more cautious, cunning, and calculating. Without the field commander, however, the strategist is powerless. Indeed, without first- and third-chakra types who are willing to actualize their visions, fifth-chakra types risk becoming irrelevant. They may be able to weave the vision and tell others what to do; but it is the "doers" who carry out their plans.

Because Speakers are mainly interested in the grand vision, they are not very grounded and practical. They have their heads in the clouds. They like telling people what could be, but don't like actually making it happen. In terms of the chakra system, this makes sense. The higher we go along the chakras, the further we get from an actual connection to life. The location of the fifth chakra keeps its personality type keenly interested in influencing the world, but is quite dreamy. The changes they envision in the world tend toward the utopian; they tend to dream dreams that are bigger than life, and more abstract.

Since they don't actually like to follow through on implementing their own visions, fifth-chakra types are inclined to believe that all they need to do is provide the vision and all the rest will somehow happen by itself. In a sense, it seems as if they think they can affect reality simply through the power of intention. Because of this, they are often attracted to concepts of magical thinking, feeling that the vision they hold in their minds can "attract" a natural response from reality. In general, they are interested in any form of control over reality.

Speakers can be so dreamy that they may even feel that their visions will be fulfilled automatically, simply by virtue of having been formulated. They tend to lose touch with reality and instead are easily absorbed in their own visions, even when, in reality, they or their visions are not successful at all. Speakers never let facts confuse them.

Nonetheless, their dreaminess can be of great benefit to others. When you read a book written by a fifth type, or attend a performance or lecture, you can easily get the feeling that you have had a life-changing experience. If they are truly powerful communicators, you may even feel as if you are ready to leave your world behind and follow this new idea or vision with the same enthusiasm with which they themselves follow it.

Speakers search carefully for the precise words that will connect with people's hearts and minds, saying the right thing with the right tone at the right moment to make their listeners open up. Obviously, this can be somewhat addictive, because when they begin to see the way audiences respond to them, they want more of it. We all know musicians who stand in front of huge crowds, exclaiming, "I love you!" Of course, what they really mean is, "I love how I am able to influence you and that you open up to my influence unreservedly." It is never about the crowd; it's always about them.

Speakers are dominated by the communicating center and want to be both seen and heard. In fact, they are the most visible of all human beings. They may not be as explicitly extroverted as Artists, but they still find it essential to leave their mark on the world. For this reason, many of them like being on stage in front of a large audience. They are impressed by numbers that indicate a larger scope of influence. They love the experience of speaking out in front of an attentive crowd; in fact, these are often their most memorable moments in life.

By nature, Speakers are fluent in many "languages"—not necessarily Spanish and Turkish, but the different "languages" of businessmen, politicians, scholars, and laymen. This makes them highly adaptable to many types of listeners. Like chameleons, they take the form of their environment and change their language according to what they "read" from their audiences, cleverly recognizing what people need them to be. This can make them a bit devious. They are not transparent, so people around them, even their closest companions, may not know exactly who or what they are. People are often left wondering whether they actually have any inner being of their own—any one authentic self.

Driven by their wish to express ideas and influence people and events, fifth-chakra types are not very emotional and may even be uncaring. They are highly engaged, but mostly in the fulfillment of their own visions rather than their direct connections with those who are meant to realize their dreams. With their gaze turned to the distant horizon, they often miss what is just under their noses—human emotions in particular. Worse than that, they consider those around them to be mere vehicles or messengers for their ideas. When a fifth-chakra type has the third chakra as secondary, this tendency is amplified even more. If, on the other hand, their secondary is the fourth-chakra type, this sometimes dangerous attribute is somewhat mitigated.

The cunning nature of the fifth type draws them to the world of intrigues and conspiracies, plots and enemies. They feel as if they are surrounded by schemers who control or try to control reality. They, in turn, respond with a secretive world of their own. When encountering disappointing situations and people, they rarely react directly. For the most part, they choose a cat-like style, concealing their anger, quietly withdrawing, and looking for a new strategy. By contrast, third-chakra types, who are transparent and explicit when expressing anger, are more like barking dogs.

Speakers are driven by an intense desire to control reality. As natural-born dreamers, they cultivate visions about all aspects of life and can hardly bear a deviation caused by external circumstances or other people's ideas. Simply put, to them, it is always "my way or the highway." As frontline leaders, they find it very hard to follow someone else's authority or vision. While they are always on the lookout for new sources of ideas, they like to be inspired by their own thoughts and to remain in control of their own paths. When following another, sooner or later, they rebel.

Strengths and Gifts

Fifth-chakra types are quite enthusiastic and passionate beings. Their strong faith in their visions and dreams tends to keep them energetic and wakeful. Since they are always gazing toward a distant future, they remain optimistic. Their enthusiasm is contagious, and they are endowed with the capacity to excite others and to gather them around one grand vision.

Speakers are intensely idealistic and equipped with a deep sensitivity to injustice. With their strong ability to understand different people, they know how to build bridges and make people transcend differences and connect with one another. They are strong individuals who are capable of nonconformism, risking unpopularity while standing faithfully behind their convictions. For better or worse, they are strong-headed, opinionated, and vocal. When following their dreams, they are positively blind to disturbances and distractions, and they rarely let go. They are good at bringing ideas and visions into the light, and as such, they are often valuable consultants for people who are at a difficult point in life.

Speakers are quite diplomatic and often impress people with their charm. Though they are fully aware of their social role and never blend in completely, they are adaptable and can even be quite entertaining. Whereas other types can be quite rigid in their personality structure, fifth types are more like shape-shifters, taking on the form of their surroundings. This is because their self-identity is shaped by what they believe in. In this sense, they are flexible and able to respond to various needs and demands.

Their awareness of others' needs and desires makes Speakers comfortable partners in relationships. In this sense, they know how to make a romantic partner feel quite content. Though they are not very emotional, they know how to keep this from being a problem. In general, their adaptability enables them to adjust to any other chakra type, and they are able to avoid clashes by studying and adapting to the expectations of others.

Challenges

Fifth-chakra types are inherently ambitious—perhaps even overly ambitious. The scope of the visions they see before their mind's eye is usually far too wide for them to contain, yet they happily and unrealistically jump into them. When it comes to actualizing their dreams, they often find themselves overwhelmed by the magnitude of their own self-created future, and as a result, they become impotent and scattered, not knowing how to take the first practical step. Sometimes, they secretly or openly cultivate grandiose ideas that border on the megalomaniac, envisioning themselves as messianic figures. Their self-image can grow to a tremendous level, ignoring any gap between it and reality.

Speakers are usually experienced by others as overly intense, exhausting, and demanding. It often seems as if they simply want too much—to be recognized, to leave an impression, and, more than anything else, to get what they need from others. This makes them unable to relax for even a single moment and entraps them in an ongoing state of existential tension. They feel they must affect and control everything said or done around them. On the surface, they may appear attentive, but they only hear what they expect or hope to hear. They often don't seem to sense when a meeting should come to an end. They give others an uncomfortable sense of being manipulated and directed in an undeclared way. They seem satisfied as long as others conform to the image they carry in their minds, but as soon as you behave in a way that is outside their expectations, a painful silence spreads in the room, leaving you confused and unable to "read" them. What exactly did they mean? What did they want?

When fifth-chakra types carry a clear vision, they can become blind and forceful missionaries. Moreover, with their genius for detecting and abusing others' weak points, they can easily persuade people to follow a vision that is, in reality, based in sheer self-interest. The line separating a desire to have an impact and a dishonest egoistic need is not always clear, and this is partly why many cannot understand this type. What is going on inside this person? Who is this person? Indeed, they themselves often cannot tell the difference between an egocentric wish and an idealistic concern for the sake of the whole. This is why, when a powerful fifth-chakra type formulates an evil vision, it is bad for all of us. All dictators have the fifth chakra as either their primary or secondary type.

Another reason why people have difficulty understanding this type is that they are so adaptable that it is often impossible to tell whether they have any substantial authentic being at all. They are comfortable lying and good at doing so. Worse, they often don't even feel as if they're lying at all.

While they are generally easy-to-handle partners, fifth-chakra types often convey a disturbing and vague feeling of distance. This is primarily because they are not transparent and have something secretive about them. But it also derives from the fact that they are, before all else, married to their dreams. Emotional experience is therefore far from being the center of their lives. It is also true that, as lovers of freedom, they can be disloyal.

Shadow Self

Speakers want to make everyone submit. They want everything to happen exactly according to plan. Their greatest fear is that things will get out of hand, that someone may act too freely and spoil their perfect script. They are driven by their need to control—to make everyone follow their script. That is why I call their shadow self "the all-controlling manipulator."

When you spend time with a fifth-chakra type, you sense that they are constantly "supervising," as if directing a play. Every word you say might be the wrong word; every move you make is carefully watched. There is a thick tension in the air, because you must play your part in the script and play it well. To keep the drama on track, the director will go to great lengths to make sure that everything follows the script and goes according to plan. Beneath the surface, however, you can sense a great anxiety, since they believe that going "off script" is worse than death. Thus, while they are very proud of having a vision, a plan, their true fear is that their vision will go off-track, or their plan will not be followed exactly. This anxiety comes to the surface when they sense that something is beginning to flow in a direction other than what they have prescribed. Since they simply don't understand how this could happen, they suddenly become terribly insecure.

The reality is that Speakers, who seem so confident and committed on the surface, are actually extremely anxious, since they tend to live inside their visions and have no idea what to do in real life. They only know how to live inside their dreams and can't cope with anything that falls outside them. When their plans go awry, they are like actors without a script who are asked to improvise. They are "speechless," hoping that someone will tell them what to say. Fifth-chakra types only know the lines they have prepared, and they can only deliver them as long as everyone is doing exactly what they want.

Life, however, tends to get out of hand; it has its own script. This can put Speakers at a distinct disadvantage, and they need to cope with this kind of weakness. Unfortunately, they are inclined to cope by manipulating everyone and everything while pretending that their plan is intended to make you happy and support a shared interest. This plan, they argue, is purely altruistic—a vision driven by caring, not at all by a wish to control. They will carefully explain how it is in your best interest to comply and why the plan must unfold in a certain way. They will pretend that they care about your well-being a great deal, but one of their greatest shortcomings is that they don't really care at all and can easily become heartless. After all, they don't care about people; they care about visions. And their only way to regain control when things get out of hand is to convince others that this was part of their plan all along.

Speakers fervently try to adjust reality to their visions, never the other way around. And if manipulation doesn't turn things in their favor, their last resort is to withdraw. They simply turn inward out of sheer confusion. Not knowing what to do, they need to readjust the plan—rewrite the script. And they pretend that this "rewrite" was always a part of their vision—what they wanted all along. They silently withdraw to come up with a modified plan that they hope will work better, forgetting the original plan completely.

To tame this shadow self, Speakers must honestly admit that they are manipulators and that they are also sometimes heartless. They need to learn how to separate reality from vision, to recognize that reality is bigger than their vision, and that they need to integrate their vision into the world around them. In this way, they can become more humble. They also need to realize that they are actually in a state of anxiety all the time, and that, as a result, they hardly let anyone around them breathe.

Higher Potential and Destiny

Fifth-chakra types expose us to ideas that can change our lives. In many respects, they are our teachers, the ones who are destined to influence us and shape our minds and hearts. As such, they hold the power to open up brave new worlds, visions, and possibilities, and to show us our own horizon, not just theirs. When they succeed in this mission, they realize their full expression in the world.

The fifth type embodies the principles of charisma, influence, and leadership. They appear in our lives as a stimulating, inspiring, inflaming, and awakening force that encourages us to change, and to gather and adopt new ideas. This force drives us to look to the horizon of possibilities, where we can think of ourselves and of our future potential in far-reaching ways. They are the ones who inspire us with new ideas and widen our imaginations to encompass uncharted worlds and unfulfilled lives. They lead us out of our comfort zones, beyond the smallness of life, to a belief in change. They give us something to believe in and remind us that there is, always, a reason to dream, to think big, and to pursue an ideal.

Sometimes, we grow cynical; we lose hope and feel that little is possible. We give up and bury our dreams. But fifth-chakra types insist on showing us who we really are at our deepest core. They show us why we should believe in ourselves and in our role in the world. They convince us to give voice to our overlooked uniqueness. They instill in us a faith in our capacity for change, giving us direction and hope for a better future.

This type knows exactly which language to use to bring out our truest, most courageous selves, and to draw on our hidden potential. Through their speech, they make us follow them into a world of possibilities that expresses our own unspoken, unconscious, and longed-for dreams. They also explain to us what we do not understand. They are our translators, who pass on ideas from seemingly unfathomable sources in the clearest and most exciting way. They connect us with new dimensions of information and knowledge.

Fifth-chakra types mediate between us and contribute to a world of peace and mutual understanding. They link different cultures and worldviews, and provide us with a common language based in empathy. They make us rally around a common cause when we are diverse and alienated from one another. They construct movements and frameworks for world change, and organize scattered and arbitrary reality in the direction of a clear and promising future.

Achieving Balance

There are several lifestyle changes that fifth-chakra types can make to balance the excesses in their constitution.

» Avoid immersing yourself in dreams that are too big to contain or fulfill, so you don't become scattered and incapable of taking even one practical step. Allow yourself to dream wildly, but then take a deep breath, return to reality, and ask yourself, "What parts of this dream are close enough to my reality and truly capable of being translated into a next step?" Keep moving, step by step, and don't become paralyzed by the enormity of your own vision.

» Avoid emotional traps like the need for social recognition and admiration, or past frustrations, disappointments, and self-doubt. These can prevent your voice from flowing freely. Resist the general air of cultural cynicism that surrounds big and daring dreams and visions. Emotional therapy, speech therapy, singing, associative writing, and even silent retreats and meditation can help you get rid of dense emotions and find your finer voice.

» Make sure that your visions and dreams, as well as the way you manifest them, remain pure. Finding some higher motivation and a greater moral context for what you want to do can help you avoid narrow drives like self-interest and materialistic goals.

» Don't try to influence others too much. You can easily become aggressive, argumentative, and manipulative if you are not careful. Remember that you are here to sing your song in the most beautiful way you can and, in the same breath, to accept that not all people will necessarily sing along with you.

» Steer clear of the manipulative aspect of your power to evoke certain feelings in your listeners. Don't let your desire to influence become too forceful and devious. Trust instead that a clean and lucid message will reach people's hearts.

» Be careful with your power to win arguments and convince others. Sometimes, you can just let go. This may not be easy for you, because, as a natural-born leader, you tend to want to lead all the time—in relationships, or even in a conversation at the dinner table. Keep this tendency in check by listening to other people from time to time; be with them and just relax. Try to find specific channels for your influence and leave the other areas of life spacious and easygoing.

» Realize that people are not just carriers of ideas who exist only to accept what you have to say. Other people have their own needs and their own journeys. Learn to meet them more deeply and emotionally, and see how you can serve them with your ideas. After all, a vision is there to serve people and not the other way around—an insight that fourth-chakra types have in abundance. Surround yourself with fourth-chakra types and let yourself be supported and advised by them.

» Make sure that you are not driven by sheer anger and even hatred toward institutions or certain parts of society you are trying to improve. Recognize the irony of working for a better world by adding more negativity to it—as in "I wish all meat eaters were dead!" Anger doesn't necessarily have to turn into violence; it can also manifest as a clear stand and persistent action.

Finding Fulfillment

There are several paths fifth-chakra types can follow to fulfill the potential of their constitution.

» Your need to influence is a basic condition for your self-fulfillment. More than any other type, you may suffer a painful suffocation in your throat if, due to certain internal or external conditioning, you remain stuck in the inner domain. This can lead to a separation of your inner world from the outer world that can make you unable to reach out. Learn how to break through that separation and follow your bigger dreams.

» Trust that the influence you exert is a good thing—that there is nothing negative or corrupt about it. You are part of a shared reality, and when you don't contribute to its shaping, you remain miserable. Shake off the feeling that you don't deserve your power to change things or that you are too weak to do so.

» Lead people toward change in the best way that you can. Don't compare yourself to the rare individuals who instigated great shifts in the world, as this may paralyze you. Strive to become like them in their values, courage, nonconformism, and persistence, but don't think that if you can't lead world-shaking change, you should drop your visions altogether. Resist your tendency to immerse yourself in unrealistic visions and be content to do what you can.

» Cultivate a belief in yourself and trust in your abilities. While some Speakers don't dare to unleash their biggest dream, other Speakers need a reminder of their greater social drive and responsibility for the whole. At your deepest soul level, you exist for the world, and if you don't contribute to a bigger change, you will remain unfulfilled. We live in cynical times in which there is very little belief in big revolutions; yet cynicism is not natural for Speakers, and changes, even in this cynical era, can always happen. Sometimes it only takes one person to start a revolution. Understand that you may be this person.

» Obey that nagging voice inside you that urges you to make a difference. Realize that you don't follow your dream; you are your dream.

» Dare to give rise to one big dream. Ask yourself, "What is my ideal? What is my vision? Is my vision, in a way, everyone else's vision?" Close your eyes and envision the best world you could ever imagine. From this ideal vision, derive your own plan for action and define the role you will play in educating us all. To find your vision, look at all the existing movements in the world and consider which of them kindles your own passions.

» Understand that, because of your role as translator, you are always destined to exist in the middle between different worlds. This can be confusing at times, since most people are dedicated to just one path. But when you properly perceive your role, you will find in it your greatest task and gift.

» Ask yourself, "What would my greatest vision of reality be if I were completely fearless, unlimited, and unashamed—and also all-powerful?" Don't let yourself be limited by your own fears or others' influence. Try to resist any accumulated conditioning that may be constraining you.

» Spend time around and in organizations—both ones you create and ones you join. Organizations are a fifth-type phenomenon, composed, as they are, of people who gather under a certain idea and strive to manifest it. Find an idealistic organization, participate in the creation of one, or, if possible, establish one yourself.

» Engage in activities that transmit ideas—for example, lecturing or writing. If you are artistic, transmit your ideas through exhibitions or songs. Make use of your ability to explain things to others. You are an educator by nature, so find ways to make things clear to others.

» Seek a career on the stage, as the spokesperson for a movement, or as a lecturer. Try writing or journalism, or any activity that lets you reach wide audiences—TV host, moderator, negotiator, mediator, diplomat, copywriter, marketer, artists' manager, publisher. You will fit easily into any teaching or educating role, from coaching and guidance to classroom teaching and preaching.

» Your spiritual path as a fifth-chakra type should enable you to position yourself as the spokesperson of a system. Becoming an advocate of your path is a part of your spiritual practice. But remember that you are not on the path just to speak out about it, nor as a missionary. Make sure that you embrace your spiritual path and don't just strive to spread it to others.

» The spiritual path is a great opportunity for you to awaken your heart and develop your heart center. This is an essential key for both your greatest flowering and your balance. With your heart awake, you can never go wrong.

Are You a Fifth-Chakra Personality?

This self-test will help you evaluate the percentage of the fifth-chakra type's presence in you. Let this moment of self-evaluation be relaxed and playful. Try not to evaluate the presence of this type in relation to other types. Just consider how much you recognize fifth-chakra characteristics in your way of being, your perception of the world, and your natural and immediate inclinations. Do not try to make an intellectual judgment. Trust that something in you will effortlessly recognize itself.

If you have trouble assigning a percentage to this chakra, read each of the following statements and consider how closely you identify with them. If all your answers are 1s, you probably identify closely with the type. If all your answers are 4s, you probably don't. Use your responses to guide you in evaluating whether you belong to this personality type. Once you have assigned a percentage, write it down so you can compare it with your other self-evaluations. This will help you determine your three-part personality type.

» I love standing in the middle between different types of people, systems, approaches, and ways of life and to build bridges between them.

   1. Exactly my experience

   2. Close to my experience

   3. A little like my experience

   4. Not at all like my experience

» My deepest satisfaction is the feeling that I manage to influence the lives of many people, and even the hope that I have had an impact on their hearts and minds.

   1. Greatly identify

   2. Moderately identify

   3. Loosely identify

   4. Cannot identify at all

» I love weaving grand visions, dreaming big, and pondering unlimited possibilities—sometimes not only in relation to my own life, but also to humanity as a whole.

1. Very true

2. Quite true

3. Only partially true

4. Not at all true

» When I encounter a good idea, I "translate" it in my head into something easily explainable that can reach many people and affect their lives.

1. Always

2. Sometimes

3. Rarely

4. Never

» I experience a tremendous urge to express my inner truths, ideas, knowledge, and wisdom; I can't imagine leaving them stuck in my inner world.

1. Exactly my experience

2. Mostly my experience

3. Only on some occasions

4. I don't feel this urge

PART III

Mental-Spiritual Types

The third group of chakra personality types makes its communication with the world the most abstract. This group, which includes the sixth and seventh types, does not really experience the world directly; it meets it more as an "idea" and translates experience into abstract principles. The interests and attractions of the sixth- and seventh-chakra types are far less earthly and tangible than those of other types. Physically speaking, the mental-spiritual group corresponds with the area of the head and the brain.

CHAPTER 6

SIXTH CHAKRA

The Thinkers

The Thinkers

» *Presence in world population:* around 5 percent

» *Public domain:* academia, scientific gatherings, research, libraries, and books

» *Typically found among:* philosophers, scientists, researchers, inventors, nonfiction writers, critics

» *Dosha constitution:* pitta/vata (fire/air)

» *Dominated by:* the thinking center, mind, consciousness

» *Shadow self:* the helpless intellectual

» *Time zone:* the infinitely unknown future

» *Traditional animal:* hawk

» *Famous figures:* Pythagoras, Socrates, Plato, Issac Luria, Isaac Newton, Leonardo Da Vinci, Albert Einstein, Stephen Hawking, Sigmund Freud, Carl Jung, Immanuel Kant, Rene Descartes, Friedrich Nietzsche, Barbara McClintock, Jean-Paul Sartre, Hannah Arendt, Jiddu Krishnamurti, Daniel Kahneman, P. D. Ouspensky, Ken Wilber

The higher up on the body a chakra is located, the more abstract it becomes. The fifth type was already far more passionate about visions and dreams than about actual people and their feelings. But the sixth type introduces a whole new level of self-reflection, as it is simply in love with thoughts and ideas. This type lives in a world quite distant from the one we know.

Essence

The sixth chakra, or third eye, is located just above the meeting point of the eyebrows. It holds within it the essence of the all-organizing intelligence of the cosmos. Here, for the first time, we are dealing with an essence that cannot be found *in* nature, but rather *behind* nature. This essence cannot be shown through features of our everyday environment like volcanoes, mountains, elephants, or rivers. Rather, it consists of the hidden order and governing laws and codes that reside within nature and the cosmos as a whole.

Whether or not we believe in God, most of us acknowledge that there is some unknown organizing intelligence that gives rise to the universe according to certain laws and codes. These codes and hidden patterns and structures, which orchestrate and put in motion the whole of creation, are the essence of the sixth chakra. They are, in a sense, the "mind of God."

The sixth chakra encompasses the intelligence and perfect order that is behind it all—the inner logic that connects everything. This logic can never be fully known and revealed to us, but we can at least try to comprehend it—even if only through fragments. Peeking into the majestic and complex web of cosmic intelligence can be awe-inspiring and mind-blowing. We admire

Einstein and Newton for being able to trace perhaps one billionth of this marvelous hidden order, with its countless levels and layers. The more you attempt to understand it, the more complex and subtle you realize it to be.

What is this "mind of God"? How does "God" think? We see the end result in the form of giraffes and hippos and trees and plants—in all the objects of our experience. But we have come to realize that a tremendous intelligence holds all these molecules and cells together, gives them form, and subjects them to a natural order. The source of this intelligence and governing law is the domain that all philosophers, scientists, and thinkers strive to enter and understand. In this place, new patterns and structures of life are conceived, as well as every idea, every fundamental thought, every great philosophy, and every world-changing equation that has ever been formulated by the human mind. It is a domain that has no end, one that is utterly profound. Truly, it is an unknowable mystery.

Imagine the ecstasy it can bring to catch even one tiny glimpse of this order. This is the ecstasy that made Archimedes jump out of his bathtub and run naked into the street screaming, "Eureka!" ("I have found!") The human mind is, in fact, the only phenomenon in nature we can look to as a reflection of this sixth-chakra essence. The human mind—consciousness as the self-reflective extension of the universal riddle—is the only tool capable of exploring this mystery. Put simply, your intelligence is the only way you can contact this great intelligence.

What makes this even more exciting is that the evolution of our understanding has no end. After all the inquiry and discovery undertaken by humankind, we are still searching for and still revealing this order—which means that, every day, we can learn more. And this will be true as long as the human mind is here to question and to know.

Constitution

Sixth-chakra types are a mixture of pitta and vata (fire and air). No doubt, their main ingredient is a great fire—the fire of an intense and probing intelligence that tries to understand, aided by a strong sense of direction. In a way, sixth-chakra types are as directed as the third type, only their ambition is within the mind rather than in the world. At the same time, these personalities have a highly active vata element that can make them seriously ungrounded, distant, and detached.

Thinkers have very strong and penetrating eyes. Sixth-chakra types like Einstein, Freud, Krishnamurti, and Nietzsche all shared an intense, yet veiled and distant, gaze. They seem to look intently, but not at you. Rather than seeing you, it seems more as if they try to "understand" you, as if you were an object or a phenomenon. Their inquiring gaze is often mixed with arrogance, as this type tends to feel that they "know it all." This adds a subtle irony to their facial expressions. With this ironic look, they watch everything and everyone.

Sixth-chakra types are almost always quite thin, since they don't pay enough attention to earthly things like food—the strange things on a plate that prevent them from contemplating. Their thinness is also the result of their self-discipline and noble determination to remain unaffected and above ordinary and mediocre human experience. This determination drives them, in general, to adopt a proud and noble attitude.

Thinkers concentrate their entire energy on their overly stimulated intellect. While they are very wakeful, their physicality is not generally strong. They may even suffer from weak muscle and bone structure. This turns them into energetic minds that drag along their far less interesting and relatively feeble bodies. In the movies, we see aliens with giant heads and very thin bodies. In many ways, this is a suitable image of Thinkers as well, as they also concentrate all their energy in their heads.

Sphere of Influence

Thinkers constitute only 5 percent of the world's population. Their classical representation is the philosopher, epitomized by the well-known bronze sculpture by Auguste Rodin—the introverted person who sits in the midst of a hectic creation to contemplate and find answers deep within.

Thinkers are the great observers of life and humanity. You can find them quite easily even in childhood, as they are the children who look at other children. They sit and watch everyone else running around and playing, while feeling themselves to be almost like extraterrestrials who walk among them. They seem to be ancient souls stuck in a child's body. They watch it all with great attention, an evident over-seriousness, and a certain sense of silence. Already as children, they seem to be very silent beings, always living with questions about the mysteries of life and death and what it is all about. This keeps them quite unsettled. Their minds are restless, always doubting and questioning, always in a state of intense inquiry, always observing and drawing conclusions.

Thinkers grow up to be powerful individuals who are deeply opinionated and completely remote from the crowd and from the opinions of others. They *hate* thinking like everyone else. This aloofness makes many of them gravitate to the academic world, a good place to hide behind books and to look at the outside world with distance and arrogance. Yet even within academia, they stand out as individuals who seek their own pathways of thinking. They are the researchers who break away from conventional dogma and lead innovative research or look more deeply than others for ways to crack open the mysteries of the universe. Sometimes, their individualism drives them to rebel against academic groupthink, and they finally retire as complete recluses and lone thinkers to live within their own self-reliant mental world. They become mystical contemplatives like Socrates who create half-metaphysical half-intellectual concepts.

This type's need to understand the world sometimes leads them to natural science, where they can work to fathom the mysteries of life in the cosmos. Sometimes they are drawn to the social sciences and humanities, where they can explore society and the human psyche. They love analyzing—looking into the ways cosmic and human patterns work. First-chakra types are also interested in understanding structures. But their passion is mainly for the "how" of things—solving practical problems and understanding the mechanics of things. They want to know how cars are built and what could make them function better. By contrast, sixth-chakra types need to know the "why" of things—why things work the way they do. Einstein's famous equation, $E = mc^2$, had been formulated out of a pure interest in fathoming the laws of nature. The atomic bomb that followed was the horrible application of his theory by more practically oriented scientists.

The ultimate expression of the sixth type is near-destructive ambition—destructive not only to themselves, but also to the people around them. They need to understand *everything*. Understanding just a part of things cannot make them feel content, even if that part can be life-changing to others. They want to reach "complete wisdom." Einstein, Stephen Hawking, and American philosopher Ken Wilber, all sixth types, have kept trying to reach what they have called the "theory of everything"— one theory that explains it *all*. In a sense, they sought to make the whole universe surrender to their minds.

Einstein, arguably the greatest intellect in history, tried to do this with his unfinished "unified field theory." Interestingly, he didn't really care that he constantly failed, because, for him—as for every sixth-chakra type—it was his persistent effort to propound the theory that was the true source of meaning and ecstasy. Ken Wilber put it beautifully: "Time goes on, and today's wholes are tomorrow's parts." Today's insight, he argued, is forever a part of tomorrow's more complete understanding. This is how the sixth type views the world—as an eternal puzzle they work to complete, piece after piece. At the same time, however, this puzzle only grows and reveals more unknown depths. This type lives with a strong sense of purpose to attain a complete understanding, knowing all the while that it can never be attained.

Thinkers dedicate great attention to finding the perfect order behind everything. Through constant observation, they try to excavate some hidden structure or underlying logic to the world they live in. Freud and Jung tried to find logic in the illogical human psyche—some inner sense that hides behind our surface thoughts and mental and emotional disturbances. Socrates and Plato searched for the fundamental ideas that govern the universe. Immanuel Kant, a combination of sixth and first types, sought immutable and unaffected truths that he called *a priori* knowledge. Wherever Thinkers look, they hope to find unchangeable patterns of perfect order. To do this, they often find themselves sitting for hours, days, and weeks.

Thinkers want to map everything. They want to form models, erect ladders, and build hierarchies of development. Models—psychological, social, or spiritual—put everything in order, slicing up processes into clear and systematic stages of growth and evolution. They seek answers by building and embracing these models and hierarchies.

Sixth-chakra types are challenging thinkers. When a fifth-chakra type writes a book, it is usually entertaining, pleasurable, and communicative. The sixth type, on the other hand, usually writes books that few can understand. Their books keep you tense and feeling that you cannot fully understand—that what they have to say is "too much" for you to grasp. While, like Speakers, this type values the power of words as the main tool of the human intellect, their expression is not necessarily verbal; they can be artistic as well. Even as artists, however, they tend to take a more philosophical approach, clearly striving to reach and express a depth of perception and meaning.

Role in Human History

Historically, sixth-chakra types were the loners of the tribe. They remained indifferent to the technical management of everyday life, preferring to find some rock on which to sit and ponder. As human intelligence evolved, they dedicated their mental energy to making a far deeper use of their newfound cognitive capacities. They were the ones who defined all the principal concepts and structures of thought in all fields of knowledge. They were the authors of the Hindu Vedas and Upanishads and of the Kabbalah, the complex mystical system of Judaism. They also flourished in ancient Greece, sowing the seeds of Western philosophy, science, and logic.

As a rule, this personality is found among the developers of any kind of primary and fundamental concept. They have always been at the beginning of any chain of thought. This is why they are also defined as "idea-makers." Thinkers *create* ideas, often laying the foundations of new ideologies and schools of thought. Freud, for example, initiated modern psychology as we know it. Though many of his major ideas have been refuted, his principles served as the initial insights that led to an entire field of human inquiry.

Thinkers are destined to crack open the order of creation and the laws of the human psyche. But this role can be a thankless one. When they bring forth new concepts, they are often either strongly rejected or have minimal impact. This is because they tend to think ahead of their time, and it takes time for their radical thoughts to penetrate. But it is also because Thinkers are often ineffective at "translating" their own ideas. It is usually the wakeful and smart fifth-chakra types who pick up on those ideas and translate them into something impactful, building institutions and organizations upon them.

Worldview

The world, as seen through the eyes of a sixth type, is a mystery or a riddle that calls for thorough investigation. To them, the existence of unsolvable questions is therefore thrilling, not annoying. It is what they thrive on and why they remain so wakeful. Their one true love is wisdom—just as philosophy, by definition, is a "love of wisdom." When sixth-chakra types can share this love with others and communicate with great clarity, they can achieve a union of minds that is a source of profound happiness. To them, intimacy with others occurs when there is a moment of mutual understanding—when people attain the same insight together.

Thinkers are driven to understand what happens in the "mind of God"—to know God's thoughts, as Einstein put it. They have an intuition that the universe is full of intelligence that awaits discovery by their probing minds. Somewhere, at the edge of the universe, this complete and final understanding awaits them, and they are always on the lookout for the one key that will open all doors. This drive to know is not necessarily fueled by a desire for a satisfying and successful result. Rather, Thinkers want to understand because, when they do, they get closer to the meaning of life. For spiritual Thinkers, this is the source of their spiritual passion as well—feeling that they will be able to unite with the divine or a higher reality as soon as their limited human intelligence conceives the inconceivable.

The God of the sixth-chakra type is a creating and all-organizing intelligence that they understand by merging their own minds with it. They believe there is a divine master plan, and if they can get even some tiny glimpse of it, they will be fulfilled. That is why, even when they experience tremendous physical suffering—as in the cases of Freud, Nietzsche, Einstein, and Hawking—they don't care, as long as their minds remain lucid and capable. Their ultimate happiness is using their brains to work toward something higher and nobler, rising with it far above the trivialities of life and realizing the supreme bliss of the mind.

Thinkers' need to understand is nearly as strong as sexual desire is for other types. For them, it is sometimes a matter of life and death. They must know "the truth and nothing but the truth." In fact, they can sometimes rise so high that they forget they have legs and feet at all. Einstein could get stuck for many hours just contemplating the great wonder of the cosmos. He called this type of contemplation his "religion." He often became so absorbed in thought when on his boat that he would drift for hours and suddenly find himself in need of rescue.

What we call the "thinking center" is, to sixth-chakra types, not just thinking. The mundane act of thinking can easily be reduced to worries and calculations. Thinkers, however, use their minds quite differently. For them, the mind becomes a most precious tool rather than something to struggle against or quiet down. They feel no need to escape the mind, because they *are* the mind. Descartes expressed this perfectly in his dictum: "I think, therefore I am." In these five simple words, he captured the entire experience of the sixth personality. As a Thinker himself, he then tried to apply this principle universally, believing that the way in which he perceived the world was, in fact, reality.

Death to sixth-chakra types is just another mystery that needs to be explored and understood. In the classic *Phaedo* by Plato, Socrates holds an intense dialogue with his students while drinking deadly hemlock. Surely only a sixth type could drink a poison while busily inquiring into his feelings and reactions, and into the question of whether there is something beyond death. Yet he formulated a complete logical argument about it while in the act of dying!

Life, to Thinkers, is something to observe and study. These intense, freethinking individuals have, in many ways, come to watch the game without really wanting to play it. As scientists at heart, they perceive themselves and their lives not as intimate subjects, but as their own objects of study. When most other types experience a strong emotion, they are taken by it. Sixth-chakra types immediately want to investigate it: "What is the nature of this emotion? Why does it appear?" This makes it very easy for them to cultivate spiritual practices like "neutral witnessing." They need very little encouragement to detach themselves from reality. They have already taken the first step in meditation, which endows them with an essential silence that other types must work hard to attain. After all, they are natural-born listeners. Their minds are not busy responding.

Moreover, Thinkers are driven to interpret everything. Even when engaged in an ecstatic or spiritual experience, they immediately analyze it. For better or worse, they find it hard to experience anything without interpreting it, without immediately needing to understand it.

General Characteristics

Many of us were sixth-chakra types in childhood, during the years in which we tried to make sense of the world by asking the grown-ups around us tough questions like, "Why do people have to die?" and "Why are there poor people in the world?" Some of us experienced the joy of study for the sake of study while in college or university, attending eye-opening lectures and admiring the accumulated wisdom of humanity.

Whenever we watch scientists speak or read their books and are amazed by their genius, we get closer to the world of the sixth type. Sometimes, we even tap into the philosopher in ourselves—when we find ourselves in an unexpected philosophical conversation, when we contemplate the big questions of life, when we feel ecstatic, awake, and deep, or when we suddenly look at the whole human story from the outside, as if we were objective researchers and not mere participants in the drama.

Thinkers tend to have a tough time in childhood and adolescence, because they are unable to experience themselves as "children" and "teenagers." Although they occupy a young body, they feel somehow old inside. They almost never fit into their age group, since everyone else seems so stupid and superficial. That is why they are driven to books and to dialogue with those rare individuals who are smarter than they are. They usually feel that they are smarter than their teachers. They speak like adults, criticize like sharp-eyed journalists, and analyze everyone. This can be a confusing experience, since their childish bodies and feelings want to be a part of society, but their minds are repulsed by it and want to remain isolated from it. In terms of handling practical human life—from getting a driver's license to entering deep relationships—they grow up quite slowly. In a way, it takes them a long time to grasp exactly who and where they are.

Sixth-chakra personalities don't experience life from the inside. This, for most other types, is inconceivable. When Thinkers contemplate the world, they usually look at it from an elevated perspective. They see principles and laws more than they see actual things and people. The life that surrounds these laws and principles is only there to reflect and demonstrate them. This means that they have little regard for relationships and emotions, which naturally call for fully engaged participation in the drama.

Sixth-chakra types won't dance at a party. When they give it a try, they end up watching themselves dancing, feeling quite awkward and disliking the fact that they are following the same movements as everyone else. In general, the experience of moving their bodies too much makes very little sense to them, so they usually avoid vigorous types of sport.

Because their minds are so overloaded, Thinkers are generally slow-moving. They like routine and tend to develop a strict daily pattern. Unlike the first type, they prefer these routines simply because they don't want to think about anything worldly. They want their days to run automatically so they can immerse their minds in reflection. While their minds are quick, they rarely give immediate feedback about what they hear. As deep listeners, they need time to take things in and, of course, to think them over.

Thinkers are old-fashioned and tend to resist technology. In many ways, they are drawn to more ancient times. They are very fond of dead philosophers and love the experience of reading books. They shy away from crowds. Although they are gifted with a certain charisma, they don't like to be at the forefront of things because they are not grounded and engaged enough to handle the attention. In a sense, they are often too immersed in their own ideas to become active leaders. As academics, for example, they prefer solitary research and agree to teach, not out of passion, but out of duty.

Sixth-chakra types resist authority and any structure in which they are expected to receive, without question, some accepted dogma. When told to believe in something or someone, they ask, "Why?" They cherish and will fight to maintain their greatest pleasure, which is to doubt. This love of doubting makes them very problematic believers. They insist on relying on their own minds as a source of understanding, skeptically ensuring that they are seeing things as they are, without projections and unconscious emotional interference. They are pessimists and are horrified by optimists, who strike them as shallow and even hopeless. Their view of the world and people is pretty grim, and they tend to think badly of human nature and its potential for change.

Strengths and Gifts

Thinkers possess highly systematic scientific minds and are usually quite brilliant. They are inventive and are endowed with individualistic and unconventional ways of thinking that make them choose uncharted and daring mental pathways. They are gifted with a capacity to look at everything afresh, as if they were the first ever to inquire into a subject. Nontraditional by nature, they think "outside the box" when entering a scientific field. While other researchers may explore the accepted paradigm, they boldly dismiss this "old way of thinking" and turn to the problem that everyone is ignoring. This makes then able to develop new concepts and breakthrough ideas.

Thinkers are very curious, awake, and attentive. They are also great listeners: they will always listen to you intently and won't interrupt to tell you what they are thinking. This can make you feel that you are completely accepted and understood. They are exceptionally perceptive and observant, and tend to understand things much more quickly than any other type. In general, of all the seven types, they are the most profound.

Challenges

Because they live only in their heads, this type tends to forget all about the real world. That is why they need grounded beings around them who can actually think of small details. One of the most obvious worldly elements they tend to forget about is their own bodies, from which they can too easily detach. This physical detachment leads them to suffer all kinds of psychosomatic and chronic diseases. They are also at risk of mental burnout because of their overthinking. Unfortunately, Thinkers tend to wear their lack of grounding as a badge of honor. They deeply believe that they are not meant to burden their minds with mundane concerns, so they try to ignore trivialities like financial concerns and housekeeping and remain busy with what "really matters."

Their generally impressive insistence on being original can turn into pure stubbornness and rigidity when they insist on doing everything by themselves and not learning from anyone, even if this might keep them stuck in a rut. Moreover, although Thinkers may start out as fully awake rebels who question all dogma, they can sometimes become even more rigid than the dogmas they criticized in the past. Their obsession with being their own source of insight can prevent them from reaching out and listening to whatever support they are being offered.

Sixth types are proudly judgmental and critical. They look down on all other types and see everyone else as wrong. (Fortunately, they are usually reserved enough not to tell others exactly what they think of them.) They are painfully rigid; whatever theory they hold is doubtless "real." They draw final conclusions about the world, and they don't like evidence that may refute them. They are so obsessed with interpreting actions and behaviors that they do not see much of the people behind them. Because they are naturally quick-thinking, they criticize everyone else for not sharing the same capacity. This makes them impatient with those who are slower than they are. They only measure people according to their level of intelligence—although this may be balanced by the fact that they also turn this demand for clarity and perfectionism toward themselves. Sometimes they enjoy being misunderstood, because that means they are superior in intelligence.

Thinkers are quite uninterested in human emotions. Honestly, they don't even understand what human emotions *are*. Because they are unable to enter fully into experience, they tend to think that, if they *think* about experience, that is sufficient. They are quite isolated—not because they cannot find company, but simply because they don't like company. They can easily get stuck in a small room without stimulation for days on end.

Thinkers are married primarily to their ideas; their children are their thoughts. For this reason, they do not engage sufficiently in relationships. Thanks to their noble being and depth of intellect, however, they usually get a lot of respect from family and friends, who look up to them as authority figures. Surely, their greatest shortcoming—the one that they constantly wish to overlook—is that it is not enough to observe and to think of life as an objective phenomenon. Life and love can be known and experienced only from the inside.

Shadow Self

Thinkers tend to resist their own humanity. They all share an acute sense of not belonging to the human experience. Not only do they avoid human experience, they just don't understand it at all. They keep trying to understand; they look into it as deeply as possible. But because they are, at heart, observers, they can never get inside it enough to understand it. By its very nature, the human experience demands direct engagement and involvement. It is the human *experience,* after all. So those who do not enter it cannot ever know what it is. They can only stand outside it scratching their heads and wondering, "What is this all about?" That is why I call this shadow self "the helpless intellectual."

The biggest problem for Thinkers is that they never want to get their hands dirty. They want to remain forever elegant. That is why they look at everything with interest, yet refuse to enter relationships and deal with the small and nagging details of life. Life seems far too detailed to them and so beneath their "dignity." Their reaction to human experience is one of near disgust. Their disgust is not complete, however, and they find themselves torn between two impulses. On the one hand, they are repulsed by life; on the other hand, they want to belong. These impulses are mutually exclusive, of course, so they find themselves helplessly stuck between two worlds.

The price of belonging to the human experience is getting your hands dirty. This is what makes us human. Because Thinkers are generally unwilling to pay this price, they remain hovering between the world of pure intellect and the world of human experience. They don't feel comfortable in life because they honestly don't know what to do with it. They don't feel that they can handle human life at all. Emotions and relationships leave them with a great sense of helplessness. They feel incompetent, and this keeps them in a state of insecurity and avoidance.

Sixth-chakra types cope with this insecurity by analyzing everything. They put a wall between themselves and reality, and, through that wall, try to understand it. Einstein, for example, was honest enough to admit that whenever he encountered personal troubles—turbulent relationships or intense emotions—he immediately escaped into science. Feeling that science was utterly pure and perfect while human relationships were complicated and messy, he chose to flee to that clean space.

Sixth-chakra types think that they engage with life when they analyze and understand everything about it. However, they really only engage with a part of their being—their intellect. And of course, they take great pride in their detachment because it makes them feel special and superior to those who are mired in the swamp of human life.

Thinkers try to hide behind books, theories, and rationalizations. They marshal intellectual arguments against anyone who tries to draw them out, and they usually win, since no one is as smart as they are. They compensate for their inability to engage with self-importance, arrogance, and criticism. They criticize everything and everyone. The truth is, however, that they are also jealous of those they disdain, because, deep down, they *want* to be human, to engage, and to feel like an organic part of life. Yet they carefully hide this desire and are haunted by their failed attempts to belong to the human world and society. To make it worse, they can't understand why they are being rejected and pushed away.

To mitigate the effects of their shadow self, Thinkers must recognize that they come to the world with fragile roots, as if without legs. They need to acknowledge that they don't really stand on solid ground—that they are just heads resting on a feeble structure. They need to acknowledge that they want to belong and accept that they have weaknesses just like everyone else. They simply have to get their hands dirty—to engage in experience and recognize that even they have emotions. Understanding the human experience is not enough. You cannot think it away; you have to immerse yourself in it. Nietzsche solved this problem with what he called "eternal recurrence"—an agreement to remain in one lifetime for eternity, without any hope of escape.

Higher Potential and Destiny

Sixth-chakra types are the greatest teachers in the world on the ecstasy of learning. They show us how our thinking center can be more than a source of troubling thoughts. The mind is a blessing, they teach us, not a curse. It only appears to be a curse because we do not know how to use it properly. A proper use of the mind, guided by a true love of wisdom and a thirst for understanding, is indeed a happy and satisfying pathway in human life.

Thinkers awaken in us all the feeling that just as our throats feel thirst, so minds thirst after clarity, brilliance, and insight. They remind us that it is beautiful to inquire, to contemplate, to observe, and to study. Many people don't know the sense of wakefulness that active and engaged thinking can bring about. Sometimes, they avoid it because they associate knowledge with their school or university days, which were not necessarily guided by exhilarating teachers. Thinkers teach us how to harness the forces of our intellect for the sake of a higher thinking.

Sixth-chakra types are the representatives of true depth—of the capacity to look into something deeply and unveil its hidden and unknown layers. They tell us that if we engage our minds, hearts, and bodies in a desire for a complete understanding of something, sooner or later the flower of life's mystery will open up before our mind's eye. They inspire us to question and doubt freely and independently—to feel driven to find answers through our own intellects. They endow us with the confidence that we can actually look for and find answers by ourselves. We can trust that our minds hold within them higher capacities and that they can be their own source of wisdom. For this to happen, they tell us, we must learn how to think consciously and not just automatically. We must activate our minds, be wakeful, and *want* to know.

The sixth type inspires us to look at life and ourselves more impersonally—not just to enter the sweeping drama of life, but also to make use of our scientific capacity to pause and consider everything from the outside in order to acquire objectivity and neutrality. They show us maps, models, and ladders of development that can guide us on our journey of growth and evolution. These models enable us to examine our experiences more consciously, and evaluate and interpret them in the right context. They keep us from getting stuck on the way and help us recognize that there is always more to add to our understanding and depth. There is always a bigger truth, a deeper insight, and a more wholesome perception.

Finally, Thinkers remind us that, above our heads, the great cosmic riddle hangs, waiting to be solved. We cannot just live our lives without at least trying to discover the mystery of life and death. We are all "cosmic investigators," and when we are urged to know ourselves and to grow in awareness and knowledge, we come into contact with the all-organizing intelligence behind it all.

Achieving Balance

There are several lifestyle changes that sixth-chakra types can make to balance the excesses in their constitution.

> » Make sure that you live around at least one grounded and settled person—someone who effortlessly takes care of details. Otherwise, you may just drift away, like Einstein in his boat. When you become too immersed in thought, you may even need to be reminded to eat, to leave your

room, or to move around a bit. Try doing the unthinkable—don't think.

» It can help you to have first-chakra types as partners, friends, or supportive family members to balance your earth element. Second-chakra types can remind you not to be too serious; fourth-chakra types may help to cool you down. Naturally, these types can easily get on your nerves as well, precisely because they represent forces contradictory to your own. You have to agree to get off your high horse and accept that there are things that you cannot understand and fully perceive.

» Try to moderate your tendency toward mental burnout; don't "think yourself to death." Pay attention to your mental balance and make sure that you leave enough time for nonthinking activities.

» Stay in touch with nature—forests, rivers, and lakes in particular. Appreciate the perfect order and harmony that nature reflects. This can inspire you to attain effortless insights. Nature, as a "thoughtless" domain, also has a cooling aspect that can relax your mind. Dimly lit rooms and music can also help balance you, although to a lesser extent.

» Seek out situations and environments that involve humor and physical movement—activities like swimming and running, sexual acts, and socializing. Although you may want to avoid these situations, remember that, for you, maintaining first- and second-chakra health is extremely important, since you tend not to feel the ground beneath your feet.

» Try to experience things without interpreting or understanding them. For instance, experience an emotional state without giving in to the immediate urge to analyze it.

» Your greatest challenge is arrogance. To balance this, cultivate humility. Don't fall into the trap of believing that your quick mind and deep understanding makes you superior to others.

» Don't take pleasure in being misunderstood. Admit that everything you say can probably be said in simpler words. Stop trying to be amazingly brilliant all the time. Try to express your thoughts in a way others can understand so you can communicate with them.

» Practice being nonjudgmental. Resist your need to think critically all the time. Once you reach what you perceive as the "truth," you have a tendency to negate all other thoughts. Learn to respect human emotions and limit your criticisms to ideas rather than criticizing people.

Finding Fulfillment

There are several paths sixth-chakra types can follow to fulfill the potential of their constitution.

» Make sure you have enough quiet and uninterrupted time alone; spend time with yourself. This includes staying away from any human thought or influence. Give yourself time to listen to yourself, to get intimate with your mind and to take a distant perspective to deeply understand. Walking silently or writing can help you do this.

» Don't spend too much time in crowded places. You feel a natural repulsion toward these places, so obey your instincts and try not to blend in too much just because others think it is a good idea.

» Allow yourself the joy of philosophy and encountering higher minds—through reading books, studying models of development, or being inspired by different systems of thought. You need systematic thinking and perfect clarity to feed your need for intelligent order.

» Make sure that any study or professional training you enter activates your central impulse to observe. Writing, for example, demands an outsider's point of view. Academic careers offer the ideal opportunity for laboratory or scientific research. Even library work, which keeps you surrounded by books, may be a good fit for you.

» It is unbalancing and agitating for you to work with people all the time, so seek out activities that do not bring you into direct contact with others. Make sure you have time and distance to observe and not be overwhelmed. Create a spacious framework around yourself so you have a space for inquiry. Give yourself opportunities to take a critical view and even perhaps to rebel.

» Immerse yourself in developing and synthesizing new ideas. Don't try to be an Achiever or pretend that you are a Speaker, as this will only frustrate you. Develop concepts that inspire others to take them on. Fifth-chakra types are usually the quickest to pick up on ideas—and, to a lesser extent, third-chakra types.

» Your spiritual path is, without a doubt, the path of wisdom—like the Jnana yoga tradition. Seek out a path of self-inquiry, contemplation, and scriptures that is founded on a serious system of thought that impresses you. Identify highly intelligent teachers who are mind-challenging and wakeful and do not demand submission to dogma. Look for teachers who inspire you rather than teachers who try to convince you, since the highest call of your soul is that you must, at all costs, be your own authority.

» Choose an individualist spiritual path. Create your own space to develop rather than trying to enter fixed frameworks and rigid systems. You need room for doubt on your journey—a chance to think things over and rebel against accepted ideas, including your own ways of thinking. You are not meant to become a passive believer in any system. Your God, if you accept a God at all, is consciousness, infinite intelligence, and the mystery of the universe.

» Pursue some active type of meditation, since it is natural for you to remain wakeful. Silent meditation with your eyes closed will not satisfy you, as your spirituality requires observation and inquiry. Avoid repetitive meditations that rely on the absence of intellectual stimulation. They will bore you. As soon as you understand a principle, you want to move on, which makes mantras and traditional practices inappropriate for you.

» To make your path complete, include compassion and service in your journey. The tendency to isolate and individualize yourself is strong in you, so don't neglect opportunities to develop balancing qualities. Let spiritual experiences and silence without interpretation be a part of the program from time to time, but not to the exclusion of other experiences.

Are You a Sixth-Chakra Personality?

This self-test will help you evaluate the percentage of the sixth-chakra type's presence in you. Let this moment of self-evaluation be relaxed and playful. Try not to evaluate the presence of this type in relation to other types. Just consider how much you recognize the Thinker in your way of being, your perception of the world, and your natural and immediate inclinations. Do not try to make an intellectual judgment. Trust that something in you will effortlessly recognize itself.

If you have trouble assigning a percentage to this chakra type, read each of the following statements and questions and consider how closely you identify with them. If all your answers are 1s, you probably identify closely with the type. If all your answers are 4s, you probably don't. Use your responses to guide you in evaluating whether you belong to this type. Once you have assigned a percentage, write it down so you can compare it with your other self-evaluations. This will help you determine your three-part personality type.

» The world is a space of endless learning and knowledge, and our role in it is to stretch our intelligence and understanding as much as possible.

1. Greatly identify

2. Moderately identify

3. Loosely identify

4. Cannot identify at all

» The best way to spend time is to . . .

1. Delve for long hours into a book by a great philosopher

2. Engage in a deep dialogue with a wise person

3. Take a long walk with a good friend in beautiful surroundings

4. Be with and enjoy my family

» Since childhood, my main connection with the world has been through . . .

1. Observation

2. Curiosity

3. Search for happiness

4. Strong feelings

» When an overwhelming emotion arises in me, I immediately investigate it as a scientist.

1. Exactly my tendency

2. Quite accurate

3. Somewhat true

4. Very far from my experience

» What would you say is the most active part in you?

1. Mind and intellect

2. Will and ambition

3. Body and feelings

4. Emotions

CHAPTER 7

SEVENTH CHAKRA
The Yogis

The Yogis

» **Presence in world population:** around 1 percent

» **Public domain:** churches, monasteries, secret orders, sects, ashrams, caves, religious and spiritual communities, meditation gatherings and festivals

» **Typically found among:** mystics, saints, priests, monks, nuns, contemplatives, ascetics, yogis, shamans, renunciates, sadhus, sorcerers, spiritual masters

» **Dosha constitution:** vata (air)

» **Dominated by:** the spiritual center, core of being

» **Shadow self:** the anti-life meditator

» **Time zone:** the eternal

» **Traditional animal:** none, symbolized by the enlightened being

» **Famous figures:** Gautama the Buddha, Adi Shankara, Mahavira, Simeon Bar Yochai, Antony of Lerins, Mary of Egypt, Benedict of Nursia, Baal Shem Tov, San Giulio, Lahiri Mahasaya, Babaji, Ramakrishna, Ramana Maharshi, Anandamayi Ma, Meher Baba, Nisargadatta Maharaj, Sai Baba of Shirdi, Bhagwan Nityananda, Bernadette Roberts, Ajja, Mooji, Adyashanti

At the top of the chakra chain is the seventh personality type. Just as the seventh chakra is the culmination of the chakra system, these individuals are the rarest type on earth, and also the furthest from any familiar human activity. Visiting their sphere is, both literally and metaphorically, like reaching the top of the world, where the very definition and experience of "personality" are vague and insubstantial. In this domain, you can already breathe the air of another world that is both close to and distant from yours. Nonetheless, this 1 percent has left a tremendous mark on human culture, deeply influencing all the other six types.

The seventh personality is the second within the mental-spiritual group, which makes its communication with the world the most abstract. The sixth type has an idea-based perception of the world, but this still includes a keen inquiry into life and the cosmos that, compared to the seventh's spiritual center, seems almost earthly and grounded. The difference between the two can be understood most easily as the difference between thinking and spirituality. Both are linked to refined cognition and introverted activity, but the first is intellectual while the second is purely meditative.

Essence

Unlike the other six essences, the crown chakra's essence is not a force that makes the world or the cosmos manifest. This chakra, located at the top of the head, holds within it the magnetic force that pulls everything back toward the center of the cosmos, or the source of all things. In other words, it draws all *objects* toward the one ultimate *subject.*

This magnetic force drives us to return to the original state that existed before creation came into being—to the very beginning of time, where perfect harmony, order, and unity were a natural state.

That is why following the direction of this force, at times of deep meditation, makes us lose interest in the objective world, as it pulls us inward to the world of being without an object. This essence is the polar opposite of the first-chakra essence. The first chakra was all about structure and form—the chakra of pure object. The seventh is the original state of pure subject.

We are drawn by this force to the timeless, unchanging, and formless state that is the ground of being. Buddhists named this essence "emptiness" or "nothingness." It is an eternal and infinite space that holds all objects, yet is, in itself, empty—like a container from which everything emerges and into which everything dissolves. We can also think of it as a dark, endless space that is indifferent to the objects that float in it and that is so infinite that even if you gathered all objects together, they would still be a speck of dust relative to it. This dark, infinite space is the background of all life. In the same way that we can see a painting thanks only to the canvas on which it is painted or hear a sound only in relation to a background of silence, we are aware of objects only because they appear within this space.

Try to feel how this force pulls you to the center from which all movement and activity unfold. No movement can change this space. It remains neutral, allowing everything and, at the same time, remaining forever undisturbed by any content. Dinosaurs may come and go, horrific world wars may happen, and the sun may even die out one day. Yet, this still center remains, judging none of its objects as good or bad, since it has nothing to do with the world of opposites. Spiritual masters say that just as we are pulled toward life, so its opposite throbs in us consciously or unconsciously—a longing to return to an inseparable and indivisible state, almost like a wish to return to the womb.

Any room is just a space with objects in it. Our object-oriented senses, however, tend to notice only the objects and ignore the vast gaps between them. The seventh essence can be symbolized by these vast spaces—the infinite sky above us that never takes shape, the vastness of the ocean, even the center of the galaxy and black holes. It is the center, ground, source, and container of everything imaginable.

Constitution

The seventh-chakra type is purely vata, the air element, with no restraining or balancing forces. And just as first types, who are purely kapha (earth), are by constitution overly grounded, seventh-chakra types are intensely ungrounded.

Knowing this, we can easily imagine what seventh-chakra types will be like. As pure space, they are energetically cool, like the deep dark of night in which no sound and no activity occurs. They are like helium balloons without a string—they tend to remain distant and aloof "up there." They don't even observe as sixth-chakra types do. From their unique perspective, there is really nothing to observe, so they remain detached from everything and uninterested in the world of objects.

Yogis are almost always very thin, due to their intense disregard for food and a natural feeling of fullness. They have an airy-looking structure and they seem quite fragile. They tend to have a veiled, distant, and uninvolved gaze, as if they are in their own world and do not share ours at all. Their entire being and expression is that of a renunciate. They are mostly calm, since they have a very cool type of energy. While this coolness makes them pleasant to be around, it can also make them quite cold. They lack the fourth and first types' pleasant, warm energy, and there is always distance between them and others because they are not really fully here.

Sphere of Influence

The seventh type constitutes only 1 percent of the world's population, for the simple reason that most people are interested in the world they live in. Very few are as dispassionate as Yogis or have their passion so intensely turned to inner worlds. In fact, even many great spiritual masters who teach renunciation still belong to more actively engaged types. This type includes any kind of natural-born renunciate or monk within any culture or nation. Accordingly, they are most commonly found among those who seem naturally destined for monastic life and are usually drawn to separate from the busy human world at an early age.

Since Yogis tend to seek paths that honor their need to give maximum attention to inner experience, they are often found in monasteries, orders, churches, or ashrams. They gravitate toward supportive environments that allow them to follow their natural inclination, which is to turn their gaze inward to meditate, devote themselves to God, or research the subtle and mystical domains. This makes them stand out even among other monks. Many monks are Builders, Caretakers, or Speakers at heart, but Yogis are the most pious and introverted among them and are not even interested in the matters of their own sacred institutions. Though they are, more than anything else, a clear representation of the otherworldly spirit within the world of time and space, their 1 percent includes many impressive figures, among them a long list of saints from all traditions.

I chose the image of the Yogi to represent this type simply because renunciates are significantly more welcome in the Eastern world—and in the Hindu and Buddhist traditions in particular. Eastern traditions tend to honor these natural-born recluses, and they are not considered a bewildering phenomenon that goes against the general culture. Eastern traditions look up to perfect seventh-type paragons like Gautama the Buddha, Mahavira, and, more recently, Ramana Maharshi, Nisargadatta Maharaj, Bhagwan Nityananda, Meher Baba, and Anandamayi Ma. Indian *sadhus*—saintly figures who leave everything behind, renounce all possessions, and wander the earth, often completely naked—are the archetype of this personality. There are also plenty of examples of this type in the Western world, however, from Christian mystics to Jewish rabbis, who were and are just as ungrounded and spacey as their fellow saints in the East.

We may never hear of the majority of these people who have appeared throughout the ages, because they don't seek to be known. When they shy away from the protective enclaves of monasteries or ashrams, they simply lose contact with the human world altogether, residing in some cave, or deep within the forest, or in high and remote refuges in the mountains. They are quite uninterested in leaving any mark on human culture, since they don't have a strong enough link to earthly life and all that is considered accomplishment in it. When they do become known, it is only because other, more world-oriented types made them famous.

These spiritual teachers tend to be responsive only to their students (who often find them by chance) and are not usually self-promoting. They frequently enter long *samadhi*, or fasting periods. They live simply and even poorly, speak only a little, and are not deeply engaged in teaching, even if they have a large following. Sometimes, they are found within hidden sects and secret orders—like the Pythagoreans or the Essenes, who followed a communal life dedicated to asceticism, poverty, and daily immersion.

Since seventh-chakra types are most enthusiastic about studying the subjective domains and the subtler states of consciousness, they can also be found among mystics and contemplatives who dedicate their lives to mapping the inner world and distinguishing various methods of spiritual refinement. Their meditation is patient and thorough, and they remain aware of subtleties of perception and energy with the same sensitivity that a scientist would have toward the objective world. Their interest in the inner domains may also lead them to a deep passion for communication and collaboration with invisible forces. This passion may guide them to become priests and priestesses, sorcerers, or shamans who use psychoactive substances or unusual techniques like talking to spirits, undergoing initiations, or searching for uncharted territories within themselves. These are all examples of their thirst for inner journeys.

In the far less supportive environment of Western society, completely outside any religious or spiritual framework, this type sometimes turns their living spaces into metaphorical caves, rarely coming out and remaining deeply absorbed in their own world. From a psychological point of view, they may seem like dysfunctional escapists, but if they had been born in more sympathetic surroundings, they might have been considered saints or at least have been welcomed as inhabitants of an ashram. Instead, they find themselves somehow stuck in a strange society, unable to define, even to themselves, the source of their inadequacy. Since they do not share the essential reality in which everyone else naturally lives, their families and friends often criticize them for refusing to cope with what they perceive as "real life."

Role in Human History

Historically, Yogis have been the ones who brought the very concept of spiritual experience and inner spiritual life into the world. They were, for example, the first *rishis*, or seers, of ancient India, who mapped the path to spiritual enlightenment, teaching methods for its attainment like meditation, mantras, breathing exercises, and *prana* work. They also inspired the writings of the profound Upanishads.

Yogis were the ones who initiated the idea that divine reality is not only a father figure whom we must obey, but also a state of consciousness within ourselves. They transmitted the principle of union with the divine, achieved through an unwavering devotion to spirit and renunciation of all worldly attachment. This revelation was expressed through seventh types who awakened the mystical heart of spiritual traditions and gave rise to small yet dedicated groups of practitioners—for instance, Hinduism, Buddhism, Jewish Hasidism, Kabbala, Christianity, and Sufism.

They also brought to the world the concept of liberation, the ending of the cycle of birth and death through a total identification with our nature as pure spirit. We further owe them the creation of structures that support renunciation and spiritual devotion, like monasticism, visionary sects, long mystical lineages, and ashrams.

Worldview

The Yogis' most fundamental worldview is founded on their strong intuition that they don't belong to creation, but rather to spirit. Although they may seem to have "fallen from grace" by taking form, their true existence has always remained purely spiritual. "Heaven on earth" is, to them, not an ideal, but a reality: at heart, they have never truly left the spiritual realm.

On the other hand, they retain a sense of being distinctly separate from spirit—for the simple reason that they do momentarily have form—and this is painful to them. This awareness leads to their intense longing for and motivation to return to spirit. To them, the world seems like a huge transparent object through which they look. They don't really see it, since they are not really interested in it. They remain effortlessly incurious and consider the world a veil that needs to be drawn back in order to reveal the one true invisible and subjective world of spirit.

Their entire world is not only nonexistent, but also unimportant. Everything comes and goes; history is cyclical. But what really matters is the unchanging truth, or truths, that lie beneath all natural change. This eternal truth is always the same; it never changes and it never evolves. Yogis thus remain unmoved by global turns of fate and are as single-minded as possible. The meaning and purpose of life is found only in the inner journey, by delving into consciousness, devoting ourselves to invisible realities, and attaining spiritual enlightenment. Our task in the world is only to free ourselves from it by withdrawing all the way back along the path of becoming and eventually reaching the already perfect state of pure being. There is "nothing to do, and nowhere to go." The world is simply a space in which we appear to be separate. But this is just a mistaken perception that we must correct. The main question in life is how to live through this human experience while remaining completely unaffected by it and unattached to it. Our goal is simply to escape this world without anything "sticking to us."

For a moment, try to see life as nothing more than a divine play—an eternal game of hide-and-seek in which spirit plays with itself through myriad forms and energies, yet secretly knows that only it exists. We win this game through liberation, by realizing that no one can win, because there has only ever been one player. In this world of One, there is no substantial free will. The world is driven by greater forces and we must simply follow an already-paved trail.

Our only job in this lifetime is to devote our energy to the divine or subjective reality, and to avoid distracting trivialities as much as possible. But this should not be merely a form of engagement or occupation. We must come to this task totally focused. Obviously, the most important activity in such a life is a spiritual practice that makes possible this direct experience. To seventh-chakra types, this is not even really perceived as a "practice." Unlike more active types, who need to discipline themselves to sit quietly and turn their gaze inward, Yogis love meditation and any other withdrawn activity.

For Yogis, life is singular, and it is also simple. All the various energies "down there" are only meant to be gathered and unified for the purpose of inner travel. For them, love is not an emotion, but more like a dispassionate, radiant light that warms everyone simply because it shines where they happen to be. Death, on the other hand, is a sort of cosmic joke. There is no real death, since only the eternal is real. If anything, death is a kind of peak experience, a time of redemption in which we finally rid ourselves of the last layer of illusion.

Happiness is samadhi, a deep self-immersion, in which we get in touch with the supreme bliss of our innermost being. The expansion of consciousness, the loss of all limitation, and the rising of the life-force toward infinity are our only true sources of joy. Yogis are happiest when they feel they no longer belong to the earth's forms, but rather have reached the end of human endeavor within the world of objects and transcended all pleasures, pains, and earthly attachments. For them, there is no greater fulfillment than the sense of unchaining their being and going back "home" as fully released souls.

General Characteristics

We are all seventh-chakra types when we enjoy the nourishment of deep sleep. This means we recognize the importance of disengaging completely from the world and entering a state of uninterrupted relaxation within ourselves.

Many of us are, at least sometimes, seventh-chakra types when we are immersed in deep meditation or in any other kind of profound spiritual concentration. When we are absorbed in a state in which the world of objects seems utterly meaningless, we are relieved of all existential tensions, and feeling that our pure being alone is real, we may not even want to return. Time stops and we are carefree—released from the constant need to solve problems and tackle challenges.

We also tend to identify with the seventh type's worldview when we enter a silent retreat. At first, this kind of experience may seem scary and disorienting, but as our initial resistance is overcome, we often don't want to return to the sphere of communication. The world we have left behind becomes emptied of any significance.

We may also have felt like seventh-chakra types when touched by a spiritual teacher or a scripture, or when a profound experience filled us with a strange longing to "return home"—when we felt, all of a sudden, that we were mere passersby in this world and that we actually belong in the realm of spirit. Sometimes, we may even feel driven to renounce everything and retire to an ashram or a life of solitude. If we do not respond to this drive, it is usually because we belong to another type and the objective world is still our passion.

Seventh-chakra types share a passion for the "now" or the present moment with second-chakra types. Both have the intuition that real life is to be found in the timeless, where the beauty of pure being causes everything else to pale into insignificance. Artists are interested in the sensual "now," however—in the beauty and ecstasy captured by the senses. Yogis, on the other hand, are attracted to the "now" of withdrawing from time and the world, and of shifting to the subjective being. Dominated by the spiritual center, which guides them toward pure subjectivity, they depict a paraphrase of Descartes's dictum: "I am, therefore I am."

Yogis are drawn to a pure state. Any state that seems pristine, spotlessly empty, and endlessly refined strikes them as more "real." After all, they want to return to what they perceive as the purest state prior to all creation. Creation seems too diverse and contradictory; they want to become absorbed in space or light. That is also why they are so greatly attracted to the concept of spiritual enlightenment, in which they transcend even their own personality and lose all distinctions and attributes.

This makes them unpretentious people whose psychology is simple. They don't speak much and use only a few words to express themselves. They also don't have great ambitions, and they only have one clear vision of reality. They see and appreciate one thing and refuse to recognize paradoxes or contradictions. They care very little about deep philosophy.

When Yogis are born into a specific tradition, they simply follow it. Tell them to pray to Shiva, and they will pray only to Shiva. In this, they differ greatly from the other type in the mental-spiritual group, the Thinkers, who always have to complicate things through their constant need to question and doubt. "Why Shiva? And why do I need to pray?"

Yogis are eternally ungrounded and can easily forget themselves in long hours of self-absorption. They find their inner world so fascinating that they quickly disconnect from the outer world and get lost in it. In Eastern cultures, this tendency is usually well received. When fifteen-year-old Nepalese Ram Bahadur Bomjon indulged in endless hours, days, and months of motionless meditation, he wasn't scorned, but rather hailed as the "new Buddha." In Western society, however, excesses of this kind tend to be very unwelcome and are sometimes even considered as psychological aberrations. Western Yogis may thus feel that they have to disguise or suppress these tendencies as much as possible.

To the outside world, seventh-chakra types may seem introverted, dreamy, spacey, and nearly transparent. Yet they are deeply engaged in a rich experience of an inner world. This can keep them quite busy. They are able to meditate for hours on end without getting bored and can spend long solitary periods in nature in their timeless space, feeling that each day is like a thousand years. Silence comes naturally to them, so they never fear extended periods without communication. Since they enjoy the feeling of lightness and airiness, they are also drawn to fasting retreats.

Yogis authentically lack the tendency to take part in the world's drama, so they tend to avoid engagement and to retreat. In their way of life, they are often quite passive and even deterministic, and they rarely exert a willful intention. This causes them to have no passion for work. Since they are also unenthusiastic about acquiring possessions, they require very little money to support their way of life. Indeed, many lead a life of poverty and feel more comfortable that way.

Seventh-chakra types naturally have a low libido and battle very little with physical urges. They are also not attracted to establishing relationships with partners or with their own family unit. When they do, these relationships are surely not the center of their lives. In fact, they find it difficult to be responsible for anything. Since they shy away from complications, they do not enjoy the hardships that relationships often entail. They like being alone, and even if they share their life with someone, their inner life remains one of solitude and they frequently express a need to be left alone.

In general, seventh types are capable of easily relinquishing their desires. As a representation of the vata element, they don't cling to anything too strongly. That is why, in their highest form, they are often near-perfect saints. While others, after a long and inspiring retreat, may want to leave the world behind, Yogis are really drawn to do so and are fully capable of realizing that wish because they have very few urges, energies, and values in them that seriously compete with their urge to retire and become one with spirit.

Strengths and Gifts

Thanks to their profoundly subjective and introverted nature, this type's presence is gentle and airy. They tend to have a cooling effect on their surroundings. They are harmless beings who seldom express anger or demands. They are uncomplicated in their approach to life and in the way they handle relationships. The light and carefree approach with which they respond to events in life can be inspiring to other, more easily agitated types. Their deterministic worldview allows them to accept reality without much resistance and inner stress. Furthermore, owing to their naturally non-possessive nature, they give their companions and dear ones breathing space.

Yogis are gifted with a deep silence and need very little to cultivate it through spiritual practice and meditation. They demonstrate a high spiritual intelligence and intuitively grasp what others struggle to understand. With their capacity to let go of possessions and attachments, they are able to move rapidly along the path of self-transcendence. In addition, their silence gives them an effortless sense of harmony and unity with nature.

Challenges

Consider for a moment the experience of human life as the gradual construction of a seven-story building whose foundation is the first chakra and the penthouse the seventh. Would it be reasonable to start building the seventh floor without any infrastructure and six supporting floors below? This is clearly impossible—yet, this is exactly what the unbalanced seventh type attempts to do.

Carl Jung once wrote that neurosis is sometimes culturally determined—some people in certain cultures may be considered neurotic, while in others they may be perceived as completely normal. A so-called neurosis too often means only an inability to fit into society, since normality is measured according to accepted values. Magicians and shamans, for instance, may be highly esteemed in one culture, while in another, they may be considered freaks.

This is the case with Yogis. Living in a culture that doesn't respect spiritual inclinations brings about an inevitable clash for some seventh-chakra types. In a materialistic and secular society, they may be considered antisocial, unfit, and unwilling to contribute to the general good. They simply cannot answer Western society's expectation that we each be a clearly defined individual—strong, willful, self-reliant, engaged, and possessive. Being perceived in this light keeps many in a state of frustration and struggle. On one hand, they know they can never belong; on the other, they helplessly try to do so. They end up stuck between worlds, unsure whether they are really meant to let go of the material domain.

The way seventh-chakra types manage their external affairs is ungrounded and disoriented by nature, for the simple reason that they lack interest in them and cannot find enough energy to respond to life's challenges. They have very little enthusiasm for things like finances, work, or ambition. As a result, they begin to float in life; they become detached and incapable of managing its hard-core realities. This makes them constantly question their place in the world. And even if they resolve to face their troubles, they realize that, at the core, they don't really want to.

This is the seventh type's worst challenge—not to turn into drifters, unable to work, indifferent to the world, isolated, and intensely hypersensitive. They may try to live in a secluded way that seems antisocial and develop profound communication difficulties. In this state, they simply hover over the earth without any substantial objective reality and without any clarity or orientation. They may not even direct their energy to meditation and spiritual practice, and may only experience the negative aspects of detachment. In other words, they can become disconnected from both the world and from any transcendent existence. They may continue to ignore complicated and challenging situations and try as much as possible to overlook unpleasant realities. They always prefer to float in meditation, immersed in the lightest state imaginable. This causes them to be intensely resistant to human emotions that threaten to rob them of their peace.

This wish to remain indifferent in the face of human drama makes them quite inattentive and uncaring in personal relationships, which are inherently complicated, contradictory, and full of tiresome expectations. As a result, seventh-chakra types are not great partners. Not only do they refuse to enter conflicts (even constructive ones), they are also unhelpful and unsupportive. When things get too difficult, they just disconnect and watch the situation from afar. That is why they can only manage with partners who are both spiritual and deeply understanding. They need someone who is actually willing to give them all the space they need, while expecting nothing in return—which, of course, makes this partner some kind of saint.

Their reluctance to engage wholeheartedly in intimate relationships also makes them irresponsible and unproductive, which often compels those around them to take on the more grounding aspects of their shared life, including financial stability. Yogis can afford to be disdainful of money and other material necessities mainly because others take on that responsibility for them. As a result of their powerlessness in the face of life's demands and their dependency on others, they may experience anxiety and depression. The feeling that they cannot manage, mixed with a failed attempt to become a part of the world, may lead them to a growing inner tension that only pushes them further from the quietude they seek.

When Yogis enter states or periods of deep meditation, they easily become ungrounded as their vata element is activated. The result is that they grow even more dependent, vulnerable, hypersensitive, and irresponsible. When they cultivate the fantasy of retiring to some monastic life, they tend to neglect the fact that, even in a life of renunciation, they will be expected to take on responsibilities and duties, once again making them face their tendency to be ungrounded and irresponsible.

This lack of grounding also leads them to a rejection of the body. When it comes to their physical bodies, they are nearly disassociated from them. To a certain extent, they find it odd that they need to reside in a body at all, and they generally prefer to correct this "error" and achieve a bodiless state. For this reason, they try to "forget" that they are in a body at all.

The edifying image of a monk or sadhu who has renounced all earthly possessions does not necessarily portray someone who is a spiritually impressive being. These figures are often prone to spiritual arrogance for having accomplished such a high degree of dispassion, and they require recognition for their "specialness." In truth, however, they often have achieved only a limited understanding of spiritual truths and are basking in knowledge based mainly on superstitions.

Shadow Self

Yogis resist all existence—not just human existence. They don't want to feel anything, or know anything, or even *be* anything. In other words, they want to evaporate—which means that, at least to a certain degree, they would prefer to die. For them, life itself is a disturbance and they themselves are entirely superfluous. They deny their entire experience in a physical body and seem to want to return to a state in which nothing happens and no development is needed. For them, meditation is, psychologically speaking, a near-death experience—a kind of suicidal escape. In reality, they have an aversion to anything that is alive, including themselves, as if all life were merely an unnecessary container for their pure being. This is why I call this shadow self "the anti-life meditator."

In a sense, Yogis are driven by a morbid desire to feel and be ultimately "untouched." Sixth-chakra types want to keep their hands clean; seventh-chakra types don't want hands at all. They want to remain light and airy, like a feather, never touching the ground. This keeps them in a state of self-denial. They want to ignore all problems and believe that, in essence, nothing exists but an uninterrupted peace. They want to look through anything that comes their way as if it didn't exist at all. They avoid facing anything that has to do with life and don't even want to belong to it. They just want to disappear.

Yogis cope with these tendencies by entering even more into their inner world. Often, their meditation becomes a disguise for the fact that they simply don't want to handle anything. They just want to retire and pretend that they don't even know there is an issue to be dealt with. They try to become oblivious to life because they have a strong attraction to death. They are proud of their insubstantial natures, and don't realize that "nothingness" doesn't have to be achieved at the expense of "something-ness."

Seventh-chakra types want everyone around them to do the hard work and take care of all the details. They are adept at finding others to handle tangible issues like money and the small responsibilities of life in the world. They remain aloof from objects in general, and depend on others for their subsistence. They take pride in doing nothing and remaining completely untouched, uninterested, and dispassionate, feeling that they are beyond "all that." They experience trauma whenever life shows them hardships and when they are forced to come down and face reality themselves. This leaves them feeling helpless in the face of the burdens of life: "Why is this happening to me? I can't handle this!"

Yogis must learn to admit that a certain part of their meditative life is nothing more than a wish to avoid problems and deny that they exist. They must agree to confront life themselves, at least to a certain degree, and avoid placing all their burdens on others. It is not reasonable for them to let others support them or manage their everyday lives. In addition, they have to make peace with their bodies, and even become thankful for them as a gift, rather than a cosmic mistake. In general, they need to be more grounded and stop resisting and denying their feelings. They have to accept that, as long as they breathe, they are on earth, not in heaven. They don't have the wings of an angel; they are just human beings.

Higher Potential and Destiny

Seventh-chakra types promote the idea of an *inner* journey. They teach us that delving into the invisible domain of our own consciousness is an invaluable and complementary experience of human life. They teach about inner illumination and show us how essential it is to our deeper sanity to have an inner life. Without it, we are reduced to noisy minds and become utterly dependent on circumstances to make us happy. When we have no ground within ourselves, we have nowhere to turn when things get tough. Yogis reveal to us the importance of silence as a background to all activity, and the value of internal non-limitation as a background to life's hardships. Ultimately, they are the ones who show us that a deep and probing exploration into the subjective world leads us eventually to find "God," or the divine reality, within ourselves.

In our stress-ridden society, it is easy to appreciate the presence of the seventh-chakra type. Indeed, as a culture, we owe the very possibility of meditation as a remedy for our noisy thoughts to their influence—even if most of us will never travel as far as they do within the inner domain.

One of the most precious gifts of the seventh type is to represent for us the aspect of "stillness"—the place at the core of our being that remains forever unshaken, like the image of Lord Shiva sitting in a lotus posture for eons without change. They are naturally connected and attracted to this center, which has remained undisturbed since the beginning of time. It is the eternal in us that remains unchanged—the uncorrupted element that time, experience, and memory can never weaken or diminish.

The Yogis' gift is the Buddha smile—the gentle half-smile of the Mona Lisa—that knows the difference between that which is passing and that which is eternal. Unlike the laughter of the second type, it is a deep smile that reflects a quiet humor based in the absurdity of life in the light of eternity. The seventh type whispers in our ears that, since at the center nothing happens, it makes no sense to base our entire being in the ceaseless spinning and turbulence of the exciting yet painful human drama. Looking into a Yogi's eyes makes us realize that, in a way, nothing really matters. Whatever seems dramatic and significant to us is, from an infinite point of view, merely ridiculous.

The seventh type helps us get away from the ratrace and learn what real rest is like—in much the same way that the perspective of the old can inform the lives of the overly active and agitated young. This is not the superficial rest of deep sleep or a good massage, but rather an understanding that the other half of life is rest.

They teach us that meditation is a wonderful support and nourishment for the active life, because rest is the complementary half of every action. It thus provides us with a foundation for all activities and with a sweet fragrance of truth that follows any activity.

The seventh type teach us silence—the ability to lose interest in our thoughts and to let go of them, even if they are thoughts of some sublime spiritual philosophy. Beneath all verbal complexity, there is the great simplicity of silence. So they also teach us deep and authentic simplicity.

Yogis enjoin us not to attach ourselves to objects, people, and physical existence. They remind us that we came alone and that we will leave alone. In the interim, we must learn to cherish this essential solitude. Since, anatomically speaking, the seventh chakra resides above the six other chakras, this type pulls us upward, as if by a magnetic force, to feel the lightness and airiness of letting go and nonattachment. It focuses us on that which will remain after our own deaths. In this way, they teach us not to fear death, but rather to consider it an ecstatic self-dissolution and a gateway to eternity. Disappearing is not necessarily less beautiful than appearing. Seventh-chakra types, in a sense, show us our own ending—that which awaits us in silence after all the fuss of life has come to a standstill.

This personality type teaches all other types that what counts in the end is divine reality. This should be our center of gravity, the axis around which our entire existence revolves and toward which our being flows. Without this focus, we remain trapped in our transient lives, clinging to them while knowing that they are fading away into nothingness with every passing day. Their clear message is that our one true home is in the spirit. If we ever wish to know truth, they tell us, we must go within. Only by boldly removing all layers of superficial identity can we realize that our innermost selves conceal divinity itself. "God" has been inside us all along.

Achieving Balance

There are several lifestyle changes that seventh-chakra types can make to avoid an imbalance in their constitution.

» Learn to accept that there is a point in being in a body and experiencing a human life. If the divine source had wanted us to be pure formless beings, it wouldn't have wasted its energy creating an entire material plane. Since we can safely conclude that the existence of the physical universe is also an expression of God's will, we must honor the structure of our physical and human lives.

» Try to experience life from an objective point of view and realize that there is more than one possible perspective. Acknowledge that there are other modes of experience. The second type, for example, encourages us to enter fully into an experience and to avoid detached observation. On the other hand, the sixth type teaches us the purely objective, scientific view, which observes everything, ourselves included, as if from the outside. Seeing the entire cosmos as a mere projection of your own internal world is therefore quite limiting.

» Learn to value and act from your heart center. The human heart bridges deep spirituality and life in the world. It provides you with a reason to embody a human life, since, unlike your meditative center, it can never be indifferent to the world and is naturally involved in it. When you ignore your heart, the world can easily seem like an illusion; when you listen to it, enlightened qualities like caring, sensitivity, compassion, devotion, service, and a higher meaning enter the picture. Any practices that can awaken the heart—like the Buddhist practices of compassion and loving kindness—are crucial for balancing the over-detached seventh type.

» Make sure you are in contact with the other components of your being. Don't ignore life's fiery passion represented by the second chakra. Don't ignore the ambition and will of the third chakra. Don't ignore the wish for manifestation of the fifth, and don't ignore the discriminating wisdom of the sixth, which is vital to your well-being because of your tendency to flatten your entire worldview into a simplistic and undirected way of life. Clear distinctions can help you make more responsible choices and decisions.

» Take responsibility for something or someone, even if it is "just" a pet. Responsibility compels you to care for others and to consider small details, which can both open your heart and ground you.

» Work to restrain your vata element. Because you are governed by this element, any airy type of stimulation can make you even airier. Meditation, spiritual energy, and an ungrounded lifestyle can make you become like a helium balloon that naturally strives to rise to the heavens if you let it go. Remember that as your vata increases, you are also prone to developing hypersensitivity, with symptoms like emotional vulnerability, an inability to handle slight pressures and influences, sleep disorders, nightmares, nausea, anxiety, and more. This can make you feel as if your nervous system is wide open, exposed, and unable to filter any impression coming from the outside.

» Overcome your resistance to the very process of grounding. Deep down, you don't really want to suppress your vata element, and you may even be drawn to increasing it to feel more and more elevated. Here, once again, you must accept that you live in a world of time, space, and physicality, not in some astral world where you hover weightlessly. Your basic misconception is that any recognition of the physical world may reduce your spirituality, while this type of balancing can actually make it far stronger, more effective, and more rewarding.

» Do something to balance your vata element on a daily basis, and even more often while in intense spiritual periods. You can do this by promoting the earth element through physical practices, by enhancing the fire element of intellectual understanding, and by cultivating the water element through loving relationships.

» When it comes to physical activity, avoid choosing a vigorous type, since this does not suit your gentle constitution. Yoga asanas and rapid walking are probably a good fit for you.

» The balancing effects of your secondary and supportive chakras can add certain grounding elements that can make your spacey nature less extreme. If there are no grounding chakras in your three-type structure, compensate for it by spending time with others who belong to these types. For example, the emotional fourth, or heart, chakra strengthens qualities of caring and relating to the world. The first type evokes an awareness of the earth, the planet, and life as a whole. Honor these internal or external influences and keep them active in your life. Some complementary chakras can even support your higher spiritual goals. For instance, the path of spiritual enlightenment requires the third chakra's single-minded determination and self-discipline. It is a good practice for you to look at other types, within and without, and acknowledge how much they are needed to empower the spiritual life you so dearly cherish.

Finding Fulfillment

There are several paths seventh-chakra types can follow to fulfill the potential of their constitution.

» Understand that you don't need to try so hard to create a "self," since you cannot really have one. You may try to imitate others who seem to possess solid and well-defined selves, while you feel airy and unformed. Although it is good to have a certain degree of will, ambition, and direction, there is absolutely no need for you to invest all your energy in the grand project of self-creation. Be aware of and resist external pressures that attempt to make you become a "somebody" in the world. You will never become that formed and "serious" personality you observe in others.

» Look for ways to live in the secular and cynical society of the Western world as a seventh-chakra type. Be ready to be considered unacceptable and even "crazy," but don't internalize this perception and begin to think that there is something wrong with you. The solution is a delicate middle point.

» Understand that the difficulty you have integrating into the world around you is not caused only by fear, suppression, and avoidance, but is rather your essential structure, which you yourself must accept. Accept that living in the secular and capitalist West will never truly suit you.

» On the other hand, if you still choose to partake in this way of life, at least do so consciously, with an understanding of why it is so difficult for you. Find ways to take root in the world around you and participate in it. Embrace your choice to do something quite unnatural to you—put your feet on the ground.

» Refusing to make a conscious choice will keep you forever stuck in the middle, which is the sad predicament of most seventh types in the West. Many never really find themselves. But, if you choose to live in the West, live in the West. If, however, you don't want this way of life, move to another, more authentic life—an ashram, a monastery, or a secluded spot in nature where life is simpler. When you remain stuck in the middle, you enjoy neither your natural constitution nor the practical activities of life around you, and you spend your time fantasizing about the day when you will finally leave everything behind and retire to a fully devoted spiritual life.

» Honor your need for meditation, retreats, and periods of isolation and silence. Be sure to create a sacred atmosphere in your environment and make your home a spiritual space. This is, after all, the only way for you to achieve genuine happiness. So be sure to establish your own meditative structures carefully and thoughtfully.

» Make sure you take care of your needs, but don't look beyond them. If you remain relatively poor, that is perfectly fine. Not everyone is meant to become rich—especially seventh-chakra types.

» Since you are not interested in money or in a "career," look for easy and undemanding jobs that can fill your needs, or professions that operate within spiritual frameworks. Don't immerse yourself in intense and pressuring types of work. To flourish, you require a harmonious and quiet environment—ideally, one that effortlessly connects spirituality with livelihood. Teaching yoga or any other spiritual method, or being a part of spiritual organizations or centers are good examples. Non-spiritual kinds of work that allow you as much inner space as possible may also suit you. Gardening, for instance, is a form of silent service that honors your reclusive constitution, demands very little communication, and keeps you in communion with the similarly silent and meditative world of plants.

» Don't try to be your own manager. Even as employees, it is quite difficult to engage seventh-chakra types. As managers, they are utterly helpless. Look for work that places you under the supervision of someone who is by nature deeply grounded and who likes filling in for you in all your weaker areas.

» Never forget that your one true full-time job is devotion to the inner life, meditation, or God. Make spiritual practices your work and never be trapped in occupations that make working for money the center of your life.

» Seventh-chakra types find it difficult to get involved too deeply in relationships, so don't insist on doing so. After all, your ultimate romantic partner is the spirit inside and outside you. The best social and emotional solution for you is to take part in spiritual communities and ashrams where you can integrate into a larger collective that will support you in many other ways.

» Your spiritual path as a Yogi is truly not a "path" at all. It is your very life. Whatever practices you choose—whether meditation, powerful kundalini practices, or a total devotion to a teacher—make sure they honor your need for intensity, which can only be satisfied by long hours of practice.

» Make sure your spiritual path is wisely balanced. A purely meditative path can turn into a dangerously uncontrolled vata eruption. Be sure to temper your path with one significant ingredient, or even a few ingredients, like intellectual understanding, connection to the body, service to others, or anything that maintains the importance of a healthy material life. Being a part of a spiritual community that encourages the element of social interaction can have its own balancing effect.

» Since you are naturally traditional and value simplicity, devotional singing or reciting sacred names and mantras can also contribute to your path. Using simple koan-like and intuitive questions such as "Who am I?" as a form of inquiry can also be beneficial. Unlike Thinkers, who consider these practices dulling and even numbing, the seventh type finds practices that focus the mind on one simple element a way to communicate with the eternal and immovable.

» Finally, resist your tendency to drift into ethereal realms of the spirit. Avoid getting stuck in deeply subjective journeys, forgetting yourself in some astral world, communicating with spirits, or becoming addicted to extraordinary spiritual experiences. Remain faithful to the core of your spiritual practice—attaining mindfulness and unity with life as a whole. This can help you realize that, after all, life itself, both within and without, is divine.

Are You a Seventh-Chakra Personality?

This self-test will help you evaluate the percentage of the seventh-chakra type's presence in you. Let this moment of self-evaluation be relaxed and playful. Try not to evaluate the presence of this type in relation to other types. Just consider how much you recognize the Yogis' characteristics in your way of being, your perception of the world, and your natural and immediate inclinations. Do not try to make an intellectual judgment. Trust that something in you will effortlessly recognize itself.

If you have trouble assigning a percentage to this chakra, read each of the following statements and questions and consider how closely you identify with them. If all your answers are 1s, you probably identify closely with the type. If all your answers are 4s, you probably don't. Use your responses to guide you in evaluating whether you belong to this type. Once you have assigned a percentage, write it down so you can compare it with your other self-evaluations. This will help you determine your three-part personality type.

» The most fascinating and exciting experience in life is the inner journey.

    1. Greatly identify

    2. Moderately identify

    3. Loosely identify

    4. Cannot identify at all

» Are you considered airy, spacey, ungrounded, and detached by others?

    1. All the time

    2. Quite often

    3. Sometimes

    4. Not at all

» What would you say is the most active part in you?

    1. The spiritual center

    2. Mind and intellect

    3. Emotions

    4. Body and feelings

» I could easily see myself living for the rest of my life in a monastery, an ashram, or some secluded place in nature.

1. Definitely

2. Quite easily

3. Perhaps for a time

4. Unimaginable

» Long, closed-eye meditations feel very natural and effortless to me.

1. Yes, meditation feels like home

2. Yes, but only under certain conditions

3. Only every now and then

4. Not at all

PART IV

Applying the System

Knowing your chakra type and understanding your three-chakra personality structure can help you understand and manage the urges and attractions within yourself that can lead you to genuine fulfillment. Tracing your chakra type allows you to recognize the soul design that makes up your unique personality. The more you understand this design, the more you are able to direct it to its optimal evolution and flowering. This can keep you from getting stuck in a system or a life structure that doesn't really suit you—an unhealthy relationship, an inappropriate career, or an unconstructive spiritual practice. When you understand your chakra personality type, your most natural constitution can flow without hindrance. This knowledge helps you make the right choices. More important, it helps you feel at home within yourself and within your life. When you are aligned with your type—not only mentally, but as a daily reality—you are, existentially speaking, in the right place at the right time.

CHAPTER 8

Analyzing Your Three-Type Structure

N ow it's time to gather your three top chakra types—the ones you have come to recognize as the closest descriptions of yourself—and begin to understand them as part of your three-part structure.

Your major chakra type has probably surfaced in your self-tests as the one you have recognized as corresponding 70 to 100 percent to your personality. Reading about this type should feel almost as if you were reading a chapter about yourself. You don't have to identify with every small detail. Focus rather on identifying the way you look at the world and the center of perception from which you observe, interpret, and respond—what you notice and what you overlook; what you find meaningful and what is meaningless to you.

Your major type is simply the one that scored the highest in your process of self-evaluation. If your highest level of identification with one of the chakra types was 70 percent or greater, consider this as your major chakra type. Secondary chakra types usually score between 60 and 80 percent. But even if you have a chakra type that scored only around 50 percent, consider this your secondary chakra, as long as it is your second-highest score. Your third supportive chakra type will probably have scored between roughly 30 and 60 percent. If you have other types that scored somewhere between 30 or 40 percent, this simply means that you have been gifted with some added qualities and capacities, which is, of course, fantastic, yet irrelevant to this process.

Now write down the three chakra types that scored highest in your self-evaluation in descending order. It should look like this:

1. My major chakra type: (for example, fourth type, 95 percent)

2. My secondary chakra type: (for example, second type, 70 percent)

3. My supportive chakra type: (for example, fifth type, 50 percent)

A more visual way to illustrate this is as a circle within a circle within a circle. Place your major chakra type, which is the core of your personality, within the innermost circle, your secondary type within the second circle, and your supportive type in the outermost circle, at the periphery. This image can be helpful, because it captures the personality ripples as they flow out of your soul.

MY THREE-TYPE STRUCTURE

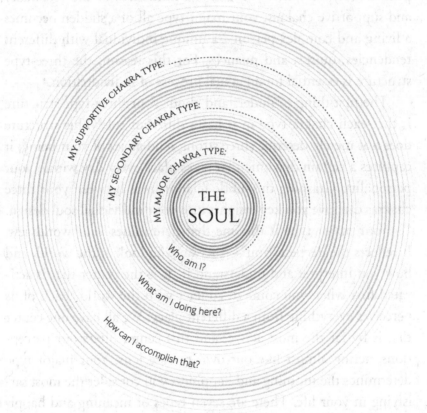

MY SUPPORTIVE CHAKRA TYPE: ....

MY SECONDARY CHAKRA TYPE: ....

MY MAJOR CHAKRA TYPE: ....

THE
SOUL

Who am I?

What am I doing here?

How can I accomplish that?

Now the obvious question is, what does all this mean?

Who, What, and How

Although your major type is clearly the most crucial factor in your personality design, without the two other lesser types, your personality would be almost like an archetype—and none of us is a pure archetype. When you add the influences of the secondary and supportive chakras, your major type all of a sudden becomes a living and complex person—a unique individual with different tendencies, quirks, and nuances. For this reason, the three-type structure is essential for an actual process of individuation.

The first thing to understand about your three-type structure is that each chakra type in it has a different role. This structure does not merely describe three strong tendencies of your being; it captures a certain dynamic that takes place every day within your personality. Grasping the subtle relationships between your three chakras can give you key insights into your individual soul design.

Your major type is the one that determines your worldview. It reflects the deepest "you"—the way you look at the world, and how you interpret and understand it. It is the center that is activated first when you come in contact with the world. Each of us perceives everything from a different place. We all have one center that is by far the most active, and this center filters our perceptions, acting almost like our own private lens. Your major type determines the meaning and happiness you consider the most satisfying in your life. There are seven types of meaning and happiness we can all enjoy and benefit from, yet only one of them grants us profound fulfillment.

Your major type gives shape not only to your worldview, but also to your "shadow self"—the central struggle and conflict of your life, your strongest inner polarity and contradiction. This shadow will probably keep you busy for the rest of your life, since it is inherent in your constitution. Just as water cannot turn into stone and fire cannot turn into water, each personality design has its own built-in constraints and opposing forces that keep it trapped in its own constitution. In fact, it is wise to let go of your ideal of becoming perfect one day, because this shadow is always present as a major catalyst for growth in your life.

Yet our struggle in life is not really what we consider to be "individual." We often think of ourselves as special—as if we have challenges that no one else can possibly share or understand. The reason for this illusion is that we compare ourselves to our friends and family, who are most likely other chakra types. But when you thoroughly study your own major type, you can identify struggles that you thought were unique to you as fundamental dissonances shared by all. If you meet another person with the same major type, after a deep and intimate talk you will probably find that you share nearly identical challenges.

Your secondary chakra type, on the other hand, determines the course of your life. It gives orientation to your major type, turning the energy of your essential personality in a certain direction. Your secondary type determines the way your major type expresses itself in the world—the way your deepest meaning should ideally be carried out. This is why the secondary type is significant to your choice of work, because it shows you how you are going to be fulfilled as a personality. Think of the difference between your major type and your secondary type as the difference between the "who" and the "what" of your personality. The "who" is, of course, your major type—the deepest "you," the core of yourself—while the "what" is your secondary type—your self's central way of expression.

Your third, or supportive, chakra type represents your top quality—the main energy that supports your personality, the central capacity that enables its flow. Since it provides you with a certain sustaining energy that empowers you, it is like the "how" of your personality.

To visualize this dynamic better, add these three questions to your list of chakras, or your three circles:

1. My major chakra type: *Who am I?*

2. My secondary chakra type: *What am I doing here?*

3. My supportive chakra type: *How can I accomplish that?*

The best metaphor for the dynamic within this three-type structure is to think of someone driving a car. The first chakra determines the purpose of the journey, the second charts the path, and the third is the vehicle that makes the journey. In this analogy, the driver of the car is the major type—the "who" of your deepest soul. The driver determines the perspective from which you will choose where to go and why. The driver has some feelings about what he or she wants to achieve on the journey—literally, what the "driving force" behind the journey is.

The path and destination are the secondary type—the "what" of the journey. It knows where you want to go and the way that can lead you there. When the driver reaches the destination, the reason for the journey will have been fulfilled. In the same way, when the soul follows the way described by the secondary chakra type, it can reach fulfilment.

The third element is the car, the supportive type, which is the "how" of the journey—the vehicle that takes the driver from the starting point to the final destination. The car represents the qualities and basic energies you need to reach your destination.

One personality who illustrates this relationship between driver, destination, and vehicle is the renowned and outrageous spiritual teacher Osho, also known as Bhagwan Shree Rajneesh. Osho had the fifth chakra as his major type, the second chakra as his secondary type, and the sixth chakra as his supportive type. The driver of his car was an immense visionary, a charismatic speaker, a revolutionary, and the guide of a generation of seekers. His path, destination, and central way of expression were grounded in a penchant for freedom, social rebellion, joy and ecstasy, unleashing the individual's natural energies, and physical liberation. His vehicle, his supportive quality, was a broad wisdom, clarity of insight, deep knowledge of the scriptures, and philosophical acumen.

The Marriage of Major and Secondary Types

When combined with a secondary type, the seven major chakra types give rise to forty-two personalities—six variations for each type. When a supportive type is added, 252 chakra types emerge. Discussing each one of these 252 types would be quite exhausting—and, fortunately, also unnecessary, since the most crucial aspect in determining your type is to understand the relationship between your major type and your secondary type.

Think of these forty-two personalities as a sort of a marriage between two types in which an alchemical process takes place. Two very different elements are brought into union, as one, they form a new type of being. To grasp just how different these elements are, think for a moment of the detailed journeys into the seven personality types we have taken in this book. In this marriage, one partner determines the way the pair views the world, while the other takes care of the way they flow together and express in the world. To demonstrate this principle, let's take a brief look at the six types of Builders we can find in the world through combination with a secondary type.

An example of a perfect marriage is the combination of the first and the second chakra types: an excellent balancing pair. The second chakra type lightens up the grounded first type. It adds humor, laughter, and adventure, making the first type less strictly law-abiding. Both types are earthly, physical, and connected to nature. Yet the result of this marriage is earthliness with a light touch to it.

When the first type marries the third, however, the combined energy is less balanced and far more enhancing. The third chakra type gives a boost of energy and ambition to the sometimes drowsy and repetitive first. Together they achieve good results in life, because they are hardworking, highly persistent, determined, and purely time-oriented. They possess a great capacity for long-term visions, and are fully concentrated on building into the future.

The first and the fourth types also strike a good balance. The fourth chakra adds sweetness and warmth to the already calm and kind nature of the first type. Both types like company, because they are "people" people. This makes them dedicated to family and community. They are loyal and lawful, not only because they want security, but also for love of communication, interaction, and emotional exchange.

The first chakra type combined with the fifth leads to a vision beyond routine. The fifth type enables the first to see the big picture and look beyond its usual narrow frame. The marriage of these types strengthens the manifestation element of the first type, intensifying the wish to build toward a better future for society and humanity as a whole. These personalities are usually good speakers and educators.

When the first chakra type unites with the sixth, the result is an excellent scientist—someone who is extremely methodical, thinks in a highly structured way, and wisely searches for general laws. This is not a grounded marriage, however, but more a fiery one. It strives for originality, which the first type alone cannot achieve.

The marriage between the first and the seventh chakra types connects heaven and earth in one personality. It is a religious combination, but one that connects laws and spirit. It deals with ways to bring the spirit to earth and how to make the earth able to reach the heavens. This personality type is earthly, yet not attached to the earth, because the seventh chakra lifts him or her with its high spirituality. This person is grounded, yet not too heavy.

Balance and Imbalance

Your secondary chakra type has a significant balancing effect on your major type. At the same time, it adds some tension and contradiction.

As a balancer, the secondary type helps make your personality less narrow. Imagine for a moment that you were *only* your major type. You would be a sort of caricature, a phenomenon so condensed that your energy would be too much for one person. Luckily, you are blessed with yet another significant chakra type that either relaxes and cools down *or* enhances and empowers your major type.

Take, for example, a second-chakra type combined with the first type as its secondary. The Artist is filled with energy, but the Builder grounds this energy and cools it down. The first type concentrates the energy of the second type and partly neutralizes it, making for a far more responsible and settled second-chakra type.

If a fourth-chakra type is combined with a seventh type, it makes for a deeper and more emotional connection to life. While the Yogi is detached by nature, the Caretaker soothes this extreme inclination by injecting warmth and humanity. On the other hand, when the overly grounded, heavy first type is balanced by the seventh type, its constitution is lightened by qualities of airiness and spirituality.

These three chakra-type combinations are clear examples of good balance. Other combinations are more subtle. A fourth-chakra type combined with a second type can result in an overflow of feelings coupled with emotions. But look deeper and you will realize that the Artist balances the overly dependent Caretaker by adding a sense of freedom and lightness. A sixth-chakra type with a secondary seventh type may seem too airy and philosophical, yet this combination makes for a Thinker who is much less "in the head," with a special type of spiritual and meditative intellect. You can think of the marriage of the major and secondary types as recipes prepared by the intelligence of nature or the cosmos—there is always some balance that is needed to make the system function and flow.

On the other hand, there is always some fundamental tension between your major type and your secondary type. They pull in different directions, so much so that, sometimes, it can feel as if your personality is split. In fact, very often, when we find ourselves torn between two opposing voices inside us, we can trace these voices back to the eternal struggle between our major and secondary chakra types.

Take, for example, a Thinker whose secondary type is a Speaker. The Thinker's nature is to avoid crowds, hide in a dimly lit room, and contemplate and develop ideas. With a Speaker nagging from within, however, this chakra type will feel torn between his or her primary nature and an opposing call for a highly engaged and exposed public role. Or think of the inner conflict of an Artist whose secondary type is a Caretaker. They will forever be torn between freedom and commitment, wild experience and a sense of responsibility. The person may not know which one of these voices to choose, since both represent highly cherished values within their inner world.

There is a solution to this tension, however. Always choose the voice of your essential, major type—your core personality. Your secondary type is only there to serve this core, so be careful not to sink into your secondary type and thus lose your center.

Your Three-Type Structure

To help you analyze your three-type chakra personality, we'll look at my own three-type structure and consider what insights it may contain:

1. My major chakra type: sixth chakra, 100 percent, Thinker

2. My secondary chakra type: fifth chakra, 70 percent, Speaker

3. My supportive chakra type: third chakra, 50 percent, Achiever

Let's look first at the underlying energetic tendency of the combination of these three chakra types. Is it generally a fiery, airy, watery, or earthly combination? "Fiery" means a lot of energy, intensity, driving force, and ambition. "Watery" is emotional, sensitive, delicate, and relating. "Earthly" is sensual, bodily, grounded, and material. "Airy" is ungrounded, transparent, detached, and spiritual. When combined, the types enhance or even aggravate one of these elements.

In this specific combination of the sixth, fifth, and third chakras, it is quite clear that these three types enhance each other's fire element. They are energetically intense types in themselves—an intense intellect, the element of leadership and speaking out, and an ambitious and developing character. Yet together, they take these tendencies to a whole new level. In the absence of any tempering first, fourth, or seventh types, this personality is not only fiery, but also highly active and "masculine."

Now let's take a closer look at the interplay of the major and secondary types—the sixth and the fifth. The Thinker is a developer of ideas, while the Speaker is an expresser of ideas. This seems to be a great connection between driver and destination—innovative ideas and theories emerge and then are channeled to the outside world. Interestingly, this has been one of the most common combinations for Thinkers who have also become teachers or speakers. The secondary fifth chakra takes the major sixth chakra out of the cave, convincing it to come out into the world to have its ideas fulfilled. This is the destination or path of fulfillment for this soul design. If this personality resists sharing its insights with the world, it will not be fulfilled.

However, there is also an inherent conflict in this combination. The driver, the sixth chakra type, prefers to remain inwardly focused—in the ivory tower of pure thinking—and dislikes the idea of coming out and being "translated," which feels rather "cheap." This type enjoys remaining unexplained and sophisticated. This leads to an inevitable clash between the two parts of the personality—a desire to communicate thoughts and ideas, and a reluctance to do so.

This problem is intensified by the fact that Thinkers don't really know how to translate their ideas into accessible forms of communication. The secondary fifth chakra will urge them to do so, yet there will always be the question of how to translate. The predominant experience of this chakra-type combination will be confusion around finding a common language in which to communicate with the "human world." This inevitably makes frustration the central emotion of this personality.

A deeper look into the combination of these three chakra types reveals one more important element. The three types, which are all future-oriented, are extremely evolutionary and driven. This can easily lead to impatience—like a race car that doesn't like to find anything in its way and resists slowing down.

Of course, this personality is not doomed to feel only frustration and impatience. This combination has some clear advantages.

This structure forms a strong individual, one who is ambitious, uncompromising, and also quite unshakeable. Such an individual is a natural-born visionary and very innovative, yet fully equipped with the capacity to give shape to and manifest their vision. The ambition inherent in this personality can be realized, since there is a corresponding ability to achieve goals. Furthermore, there is a capacity for deep understanding coupled with the skill to make sense of insights with clarity, order, and creativity.

This structure reveals a rather efficient personality—an innovative thinker, deeply driven to convey and manifest concepts, and equipped with a lot of energy to do so. However, this combination is guided by ideas and visions, and wants to scale the heights. It lacks the more human-oriented types like the first, second, and fourth to balance it. It has no cooling and relaxing element. One of the dangers for this personality type is a tendency to burn themselves out.

To balance this personality, we simply need to look to the other four chakra types that are not present in its design—in this case, the first, second, fourth, and seventh. Here are some suggestions from these types:

» From the first type: seek out ritual-like routines to provide a ground for your ever-developing system; deal with small details and practicalities; use some relaxing herbs like chamomile or mint.

» From the second type: live in soothing surroundings, next to nature—forests and lakes—or even just spend time in nature; introduce mild and enjoyable physical activity into your routine.

» From the fourth type: establish loving relationships with cooling people like fourth or seventh types, and, to a certain degree, second types. Be aware that the first type is overly opposing in balance and may clash with so much intensity.

» From the seventh type: pursue a daily meditation, preferably at a fixed time of the day.

Now let's look at your own chakra combination to derive insights for achieving a balanced and fulfilled way of life. Use the following questions as a general framework. Take your time so you can learn as much as possible from your three-type structure.

When answering questions 1 and 2, try not to be ambiguous—"It is airy, but also watery and a little fiery" or "It is masculine, but also feminine." This can keep you from reaching any significant conclusion about yourself. Strive for clear definitions. Expose excesses and imbalances, so that you can eventually come up with possible ways to achieve balance.

1. Is my design generally fiery, watery, airy, or earthly?

2. Is it more masculine or more feminine?

3. Are there balancing elements present in my personality, or do all three chakras enhance each other? Is the combination too relaxed?

4. How does my secondary chakra type contribute to my major type? How does it contradict it?

5. What is the struggle between my major and secondary chakra types?

6. What are the positive and negative emotions I feel as a result?

7. What are possible occupations for me, and how can I contribute to others?

8. What strengths can I bring to the work in which I am currently engaged? How do I struggle with it?

9. What do I need to do to balance my major and secondary chakra types?

There are general orientations for the dominant elements of each chakra type. However, in certain combinations, some of the types actually change their nature and enhance the other elements.

1. The first type, or Builders, can enhance the earth element and feminine qualities when combined with Artists, Caretakers, and Yogis. But in more masculine combinations—with Achievers, Speakers, and Thinkers—it supports the fire element and "turns" masculine.

2. The second type, or Artists, can enhance fire and masculine qualities when combined with Achievers, Speakers, and Thinkers. But in more feminine combinations—with Builders, Caretakers, and Yogis—it supports the water element and "turns" feminine.

3. The third type, Achievers, enhances fire and masculine qualities in all structures.

4. The fourth type, Caretakers, supports water or air and feminine qualities in all structures.

5. The fifth type, Speakers, enhances fire and masculine qualities in all structures.

6. The sixth type, Thinkers, supports fire and masculine qualities in all structures.

7. The seventh type, Yogis, supports air and feminine qualities in all structures.

Be intuitive when analyzing your own chakra combinations. After learning about all seven major types, you can simply look at the percentages you have assigned and feel them energetically. How do you *feel* when you look at your combination?

Just as there are no "good" or "bad" personalities, there are no good or bad chakra combinations. Any combination can be balancing and empowering, or conflicted and contradictory. Learning the three main components of your personality can help you accept your own constitution as it is. Then ask yourself, "How can I make the best out of my structure and not just accept the clashes it contains as a sort of an inherent existential state?" Any secondary chakra type can balance rather than contradict; any supportive chakra can be truly supportive.

On the other hand, we have to accept some degree of imbalance. After all, we are a dish that will forever be too spicy, too salty, too sour, or too sweet. We can never be perfectly balanced, so we must remember this law of nature: sometimes a little imbalance is a part of balance. A certain amount of friction within your system is also essential for self-development. Strive to attain an optimal balance, while making sure that your constitution doesn't harm you or others.

CHAPTER 9

Fulfilling Your
Chakra Type

You can learn a lot from the system of chakra personality
types about your potential for inner and outer peace—
about the possibility of making peace with your own self,
and about attaining peace in your relationships with others.

Inner peace is the basis of any other type of peace. When you
are at peace with yourself, you are much more capable of embracing and understanding others. This kind of self-acceptance does
not mean that you overlook the limitations and downsides of your
type. It only means that you don't focus on them more than necessary and pay a great deal of attention to the gifts and strengths
of who and what you are.

We always tend to move between two extremes—self-acceptance and the need to change and improve ourselves. When you learn about your soul design, you become acquainted with a pattern that you should accept as it is—its limitations as well as its strengths. At the same time, you also want to transcend your design, to change your patterns and limitations in order to achieve balance and find fulfillment. None of us can remain a purely individual design, since life calls us to develop other areas and dimensions in order to be whole human beings. To attain a holistic balance, we cannot ignore any of the lessons or challenges put before us by life.

This means we somehow need to learn both how to accept ourselves *and* change ourselves. However difficult, we have to keep moving between the two extremes of being just the way we are, including our limitations, and going against ourselves to break through our limitations and become a "higher me." Unconsciously, we keep asking ourselves this question: When are we meant to accept who we are and see the beauty of ourselves—the beauty of our weaknesses included—and when are we meant to seek change?

Obviously, we are not just flowers of the universe. Even if you wanted to, you couldn't completely accept your soul design. You have a mind that, for better or worse, gives you the feeling that, to a certain degree, you can change your destiny. Sometimes this is a source of great suffering, because you believe you can change and have a sense of your greater potential. Yet you may lack sufficient energy or courage to follow through on this promise. When you look at yourself through the lens of potential and condemn yourself for not being able to live up to it, you miss the point and can be lost in frustration. You must learn to relax into what you are.

How can you tell when it is time to obey the whisper of self-love that tells you to relax and accept yourself and when it is time to reject it? Is there a way to negotiate between these two extremes?

Contemplating whether your type is "nature or nurture" leads you to realize that it actually precedes both. This is because, in the deepest sense, your type is your "soul design." It is your most profound attraction and calling, carefully planned according to the purpose of your soul's journey. It is what you are meant to learn and manifest in this lifetime in order to fulfill your purpose.

That is why your soul design is crucial for the attainment of your higher form of destiny. This higher destiny is often an overlooked potential, one you cannot identify and that others do not encourage you to look for within yourself. This makes the revelation of your type an indispensable self-knowledge, since it reveals the seeds of potential that lie dormant deep inside you. When you confidently know your type, you can follow your destiny with accuracy while avoiding the pitfalls of your conditioned personality. On the basis of such an understanding, you can also more easily derive many lesser choices—like your ideal career, relationship, spiritual path, and lifestyle.

This knowledge can be suppressed by different experiences in life that may have taught you that you shouldn't listen to your soul, but rather conform. Often, your true potential is deeply buried and suppressed as a result of some social role taking the place of your soul's fulfillment. That is why this process of self-discovery is like extricating a diamond from beneath the more superficial layers of personality you may have developed over time. Finding this diamond is similar to what we sometimes consider being able to listen to our soul's deepest call.

Some of us are more naturally aligned with our soul's deepest call and thus are very close to our true type, while others have distanced themselves from this inherent calling. That is why we find such a vast range of expressions of each type, some minimal and weak, and some so extraordinary in their manifestation that they bring to the world a near-perfect embodiment of their chakra essence.

That is why I have given you the names of well-known historical figures who represent each of the types. These figures are like each type's special heroes. From their life stories, actions, and statements, we can learn what a higher manifestation of each type looks like. This can set an inspiring example for us, and show us how our own being could reach its highest potential by fully and uncompromisingly expressing our major chakra perspective.

Learning about great examples of your type can evoke in you an inspiration to raise yourself from your basic chakra type toward the heights that your innate destiny contains. Don't despair because you think these examples are too great to follow. As far as your personality type is concerned, it is not about the scope of impact you have, but rather about the degree of your loyalty to what you truly are. It is thus wiser to use these stories to indicate what it is like when your type reaches full maturation and flowering as a soul in human form.

As fully developed souls, these chakra-type heroes reveal just one face out of the seven faces of the divine or higher reality. Since the seven chakra essences comprise what can be regarded as the "multifaceted God," each type has the destiny to fulfill one facet of the diamond of divine reality. As its highest ambition, the system of the seven personalities aims at this level of self-fulfillment for all of us.

Balancing Your Type

The chakra-type system tells us that we are only meant to change our excesses. When your soul design begins to be auto-destructive—when you begin to destroy yourself, ruin your body, and become dysfunctional in life, or when you begin to destroy others around you and your relationships, this is a sure sign that you must pause and turn to changing yourself.

Luckily, we can easily tell when we are mired in excess and in a self-destructive mode. We have the best warning system we could hope for to tell us when things are unbalanced—our bodies. Our bodies are always there to remind us when we have too much fire, air, earth, or water. They speak to us through psychosomatic diseases and chronic problems—when we don't sleep well or when we sleep too well; when we barely drag ourselves out of bed in the morning and when we suffer from irritable bowel syndrome. All our excesses have immediate physical reflections.

Another clear way to know when your type is imbalanced is to observe the repetitive thoughts that drive you crazy or certain emotions that eat you up. Imbalance can also be reflected in your relationships—for example, when several people tell you the same thing.

Knowing how to stop before reaching a harmful imbalance requires true mastery—just like knowing exactly the right point to stop eating. It is wisest not to wait to reach the moment of burnout—whether emotional burnout for the fourth type, mental burnout for the sixth, or spiritual burnout for the seventh.

Of course, we can always argue that, if second-type Jim Morrison had not burned out, he wouldn't have been "Jim Morrison" at all. Surely, there is some beauty in being Jim Morrison, living between such extremes—yes, he sacrificed his life, but what a legendary life! Self-sacrifice is often admirable in our eyes precisely because it seems to accept and ignore what we consider to be "excess." Those called to lead "legendary" lives simply go all the way with their type's excesses. But if you want to learn the wisdom and art of a balanced life, you have to learn when these tendencies begin to become auto-destructive. Look back on the chapters that outlined each type to find descriptions of the points at which each type's energy begins to overflow and cause deep imbalances.

When your chakra energies prevent you from being able to live a fulfilled and balanced life, that is when you should restrain them. Other than that, we are all meant to reach a profound self-acceptance. However, we are mostly incapable of doing that. Why? For the simple reason that we don't accept our soul design in general. We feel limited by it, since there are certain behaviors and capacities we can never express. We may also feel that we are not like "others," or that we are not what we "should" be. Simply put, our *design* disturbs our *self-image*.

This has a lot to do with the society around us, which keeps telling us who and what we should be. Too often, we suppress and bury our type beneath social masks simply because we are told that the way we are is not the way we should be. Slowly but surely, we internalize this nonacceptance.

To resist this tendency, you must learn to love your soul design. Before appreciating other people's personality types, learn to appreciate and cherish your own. Sadly, for too many of us, even after reading a positive and extensive description of the gifts of our own types, we may still have some nagging feeling that there is something wrong with us. While knowing your pattern makes you acknowledge your individuality and uniqueness, it can also make you feel different and isolated.

It seems that everyone thinks all others should be exactly like them. When another person advises you to stop doing this or to start doing that, what they truly mean is, "Start being like me! If you only stopped being you and started being me, I would be so much happier!" Builders may hear "Don't sweat the small stuff. Life is too short!" while Artists may hear "Stop being so lazy. Life is not just about enjoyment." Achievers are often told to "Stop doing so much! You are a workaholic," while Caretakers are told to "Grow up! What is all this sensitivity? And why all these tears?" Speakers are warned to "Stop dreaming so big. Do only what you can and that is enough," while Thinkers are encouraged to "Stop thinking so much. Start enjoying life in the body!" And Yogis are ordered to "Stop escaping life. You are always running away."

We all hear what we should stop being or doing all the time, and this is when we begin to feel that something is wrong with us and that we had better adjust. When, for example, a fifth type is constantly told in childhood to stop dreaming and be practical, they may suppress their tendency to dream on a large scale.

Of course, all these statements are half-true, since people do point out our excesses in a kindly way as well. And when we receive loving reflections on our more destructive excesses, we should generally welcome them. However, these encouragements are only relevant when you are clearly doing something destructive to yourself or to others. Jim Morrison, for example, could have benefited from hearing, "It is wonderful that you are so wild, but please stop with the alcohol and drugs so that you can live to more than thirty!" Unfortunately, most remarks from most people are not meant to help us balance ourselves; they are intended to make us stop *being* ourselves and to start being like them. Partners and parents in particular are quite diligent at trying to shape their lovers or children in their own image.

Knowing your type can give you a profound feeling of yourself that can withstand criticism and manipulation. When you are confident of your true values, you can be more awake when you are criticized because you don't share someone else's values. You feel able to say, "No, now you are just talking from your own world. This is what you believe in, and I respect that, but I am not going to be a different person just for you."

Accepting Yourself

The first step on your path to inner and outer peace is self-acceptance, learning to love and celebrate your soul design.

We live in a society dominated by the first, third, and fifth chakra types. They run the governments and the educational systems, control the money flow, and make the laws. They define the values on which our society is founded. The first type values building, creating stability and security, contributing to the system, and being like everyone else. The third type values achieving, becoming "someone," succeeding, and reaching the top. The fifth type values self-fulfillment, free expression, and becoming your own individual, including frantically trying to "go viral" and to gain global recognition.

This type of society is not interested in cultivating our talents, but rather in making use of them. When you cultivate a talent, you don't know exactly how it will flower. But society knows exactly what direction it wants it to take. So when your talents begin to serve practical and success-oriented ends, you begin to forget who you are and what your real inclinations are, because your talents are already being directed in service to something else.

Such a society is not an ideal environment for second, fourth, sixth, or seventh types. In terms of values and a genuine space for expression, these types tend to feel completely excluded. Of course, they have their public spheres of influence—comedy clubs or academia—but the general atmosphere dictates that we all fall under the power of the first, third, and fifth types, who simply don't consider the values of the other four as being significant enough to further the progress of the social machine.

When those with these chakra types are unable to fit into their surroundings, they begin to doubt their own values and to become a type that is not their own. As a result, even while reading this book, you may not be sure what your type really is, because you may not know how to separate your authentic self from your own self-image and the external voices that are shaping you. Your personality type may be deeply buried beneath commitments and pressures, upbringing and conditioning, and sometimes even deeper karma—different forces that have made you choose and do certain things that suffocate you instead of allowing your type to flower.

This makes self-acceptance an intense process, especially for second, fourth, fifth, and seventh types, because it is difficult for them to declare their different and independent values. Naturally, not sharing the values of the general society presents a serious challenge. However, this is the lesson of self-acceptance: "I want to be like me." Remember, as long as your life doesn't follow the pattern of your type, you are like a fish out of water, struggling to swim on dry land. You must learn to relax into your own soul design, live your own values, and remain authentic—even when your family resents your type, or your partner is determined to remold you, or your workplace demands that you change. After all, this capacity is what makes you a real individual.

Feeling your major chakra type means not only recognizing it as a truth about yourself—as an accurate description of your personality—but, more deeply, feeling it as your own innate soul design: "This is what I am."

Now turn love toward this design. Love yourself as this design. Taking into account both its gifts and its limitations, tell yourself, "This is how the divine reality, life's infinite intelligence or the universe, made me—beautiful and flawed, balanced and unbalanced, and sometimes even beautiful *because* of my limitations."

We never think of one flower as being better or more important than other flowers. In this context, we are like flowers. And not accepting your own soul design is like not accepting the universe as a whole. Surrendering to your soul design means surrendering to the higher will.

It is all perfect. You are in your right design—in your right role in the universe. Remember that only when you accept yourself can you ever hope for a real flowering of the gifts inherent in your design.

Accepting Others

The second step on your path to inner and outer peace, which is necessary for achieving harmonious relationships, is to eliminate the pride of your personality type. It is rather ironic that, with all the difficulty we have accepting ourselves, every type has a tremendous sense of self-importance and superiority when it comes to its own perception of reality.

Each type looks down on all other types, thinking, "How could they miss the whole point?" Caretakers wonder why others can't understand that only love and caring matter. They believe that emotions are superior to thinking and pity those who cannot feel, are "stuck in their heads," or are too egotistic to think of others. On the other hand, Thinkers are amazed that others don't understand that intelligence and knowledge are all that matters. To them, everyone else looks stupid, superficial, overly physical, and unselfconscious. Builders are puzzled because people are so ungrounded. And Artists laugh at all three, wondering how they could be so serious and boring and miss out on the whole experience of life.

Let's just admit it. We are all quite arrogant. That is why it is not enough to free ourselves from self-rejection and allow ourselves to be who we are. We must also free others from rejection and let them be their own true selves as well. When you begin to observe the way we judge others all day long, you quickly realize that what we judge is their type. This is what we don't like about others. We scrutinize their excesses and limitations and judge them from within our own type.

Our task is, therefore, to expand the acceptance we have turned toward ourselves to include others. When we accept ourselves, we begin to feel our type as part of the complete cosmic puzzle. But this means that all others are an integral part of it as well. Rather than criticizing either ourselves or others, we must learn to use our personality as a way to highlight our own unique role, as well as the unique roles of others.

Think of one person who clearly belongs to a completely different type, someone who is intensely different from you in values and perspective. This could be anyone you know—an acquaintance, your partner, your child, a parent, a friend, a coworker, or a famous or perhaps historical figure. Take a look at this person and try to see their beauty of perception and experience. Recognize that this person's values are just as valid as your own and reflect a complete and perfect perspective on reality. Finally, think of this person as your teacher. What can this person give you that you cannot give yourself, even if you wanted to?

People, believe it or not, are really not meant to be you. There is enough "you" in the world. All of us were made by God or the universe, so if God or the universe needed other types to enter creation with a certain design, how can you prefer otherwise? What makes you think your design is better or more special?

Now try humbly approaching this person, even if only internally, and admit, "You have something I don't have." Acknowledging that someone's perspective is as complete and valuable as your own is a key to harmony in all your relationships. In reality, there is no hierarchy—those who are intelligent are not "better" than those who are joyful, and those who are joyful are not "better" than those who are loving. We are all growing as one field of flowers, and each blossom in that field is indispensable. Remember, without the influence of other types in your three-part structure, you are missing something. Humility and acceptance of others makes us capable of receiving their gifts.

Achieving Harmony

When we know how to accept ourselves and, at the same time, how to accept others' different values and gifts, we are ready to accept the entire world. As soon as we agree to remove the arrogant judgment of our type, we are ready to bring harmony to our relationships with all other types and with the world around us. The principle is simple: just study each type and then learn to focus on its gifts, not its challenges—on what others can bring to your connection with them.

Ordinarily, all the clashes we have with others occur because we are different types with different values. Try emphasizing the very same differences that make you collide as gifts and consider the possible result. In other words, learn to view the source of conflict as the key to union.

It is interesting that we almost never enter relationships with our own type. Rather, we tend to look for complementary types, for others who can complete us. This is essentially the source of human attraction—connecting with those who are truly different from us. Men and women, for example, sometimes seem to come from different planets, still they strive to unite. Apart from the obvious biological urge to do so, their attraction is caused by a feeling of mysterious "otherness." This means that, deep down, we want others to be others.

Sometimes, we observe people around us and project our tendencies and values onto them as some sort of unfulfilled potential.

We think or even tell them that they have "such great potential" to be much more loving, responsible, learned, or spiritual, according to the perspective of our type. To achieve harmony in the world, however, we must learn to remove this lens of "potential" and begin to see others *as they are*. We must focus on what others already have—their much-needed gifts to us and to all others.

This task may seem difficult only because we are not eager to take it on. Even after intellectually recognizing all the wonderful gifts of all seven types, when it comes to real life, we are put off by others' differences. We find it hard to accept that others can offer qualities we don't have.

Here are four simple yet powerful exercises that can help you overcome your reluctance to accept the gifts of others as constructive parts of your own experience. Remember, there is a great deal of conscious work that can be done between partners—from siblings to coworkers to couples—that can help you avoid many collisions and complications. For the most part, people in relationships just wait for collisions to happen and only then collaborate to develop their connection. They fail to see that the confrontation is a natural outcome of neglecting a problem that a little conscious work might have prevented.

» Sit together and make a list of all the good qualities each one naturally has that the other doesn't. This list will move the discussion from an abstract idea to a conscious recognition. From this list, develop a list of all the good qualities that your connection contains from both your types. Now consider how, together, you have formed a greater entity blessed with many qualities and capacities. To even consider your combined energies and gifts can be very empowering. Ask yourselves, "What mixture do we create? What is our 'new' personality type?"

» Now create a list of all the needs you each have. Ideally, you should each take responsibility for respecting and sometimes fulfilling the other's need. If you are a first type living with a second type, you must honor your partner's love of change; your partner must respect your need for safety. Showing that we care about each other's needs also demonstrates what true love means. Moreover, these needs can often turn into gifts. When people have an opportunity to express their needs, it can also be an opportunity for them to balance their partners. The need of the second type for more enjoyment in life can be an indirect remedy for a first type's tendency to heaviness and over-seriousness. When you let others express and live out their needs, you may be surprised to see that this eventually benefits you as well. To begin with, you will surely benefit from a happier child, friend, or partner.

» Now make a list that contains each person's excessive tendencies. Ideally, each type needs to ask the other to remind them when they suffer from this excess. Of course, this must be a mutual agreement and one that is limited to the tendencies that are contained in the list. Abusing this delicate trust by constantly pinpointing any weakness is not beneficial at all. You must also agree that, if, in real time, the other finds the help offered to be completely inappropriate, you will withdraw at once without pushing too hard. Use this list only when help is needed and only when help is welcome. At other times, remind yourself that you are with this person by choice. It doesn't make sense to complain about someone's limitations; spending time with someone while wishing they were someone else is simply not fair. Any healthy relationship needs to be based on a mutual recognition of each other's gifts. That's what relationships are for—to meet in order to empower one another.

» Now make a list of what aggravates both of you. Every combination of types creates and enhances a certain shared imbalance and excess. More than that, each partnership creates a certain shared "ego" grounded in self-importance and resentment toward others and the world at large. You may share some conflict with life or with others. Sadly, instead of helping resolve this conflict, you may only encourage each other. For instance, two personalities may enter into a relationship both feeling that they are surrounded by enemies. If they enhance each other's paranoia by cultivating the feeling that everyone is bad, they can quickly become overly critical of others instead of helping each other change this habit.

With a deep mutual understanding and conscious work, any combination of types can achieve harmony. On the other hand, relationships between matching types can fail precisely because they have taken for granted their inherent "chemistry." In the end, relationships are only what we make of them.

CONCLUSION
CHAKRAS AS A PATH TO PEACE

The discovery of your major chakra type holds within it a crucial understanding of your unique type of happiness, meaning, and focus in life. This is, perhaps, the one factor that distinguishes this system of personality analysis and self-instruction from many others. It is a system that deals, most of all, with value, meaning, and purpose—with the most fundamental longings that stem from the core of your being. It highlights your most sublime potential and your authentic role in life, as opposed to the social role you may have assumed over time.

This system is grounded in two simple principles:

» Your meaning in life is fulfilled when you come to represent the essence of your type to its fullest.

» Your happiness in life is achieved when you live according to this essence.

In other words, when you know your type, you know why you're here. When you don't live to fulfill your type, however, you may find yourself quite unhappy because you are trying so hard to be someone else—and that, of course, can never be constructive.

In fact, your true chakra type is often not what you think or want yourself to be. Sometimes it is covered up by habits, social conditioning, and self-misunderstandings that obscure your true purpose. When you don't know or can't recognize your soul design, you cannot tell exactly who you are. And without this intimate feeling of yourself, you risk putting yourself in certain places and with certain people that cannot support your right path. Social pressures, people's expectations, and spending too much time in the presence of dominant people who perceive reality's value and meaning very differently from you can lead you to abandon your true nature and become "someone else."

When you are unaware of your chakra type, you may live in the same house with another type without any mutual appreciation of the gifts you have to offer each other. If you are intolerant of each other's unique types of happiness and meaning, you may feel reluctant to listen to each other's needs and tendencies, considering them to be only excuses or escapes, or evidence of rigid habits and stubborn opinions. Many suffer in this way simply because they are unable to understand the people around them who do not share their own yearnings and inclinations—which they themselves may not fully identify with or understand. Others make the mistake of attempting to follow practices or adopt habits that seem to be applicable for all—a meditation practice touted as the "ultimate path," or a physical exercise regime considered the "latest fashion." The truth is that each type has its own set of practices that are naturally in line with their unique rhythm and flow.

Only when we understand our own unique chakra constitution can we begin to develop into whole individuals. And only when we gather all seven chakra types into one holistic structure can we begin to develop a fully functioning society—a human culture based on a harmony of forces, influences, and inspirations. All seven types are absolutely essential in any worthwhile society.

This is why understanding the chakra personality types can point us to a path of peace. It can help us recognize that all perspectives have a role to play in shaping the world and bringing harmony to our culture. Each counts as an *equal* and essential component of our reality.

Peace begins with a humility that admits that no chakra type has all the answers. It is ridiculous to look down on other types and think that you've got the one key to the mysteries of the universe and that no one else knows what they're talking about. This is precisely the source of all conflict in society, whether in personal relationships or between nations. When everyone is busy telling everyone else how and what they should be and what they should do, conflict is inevitable. These conflicts may start with small misunderstandings—like the second-chakra type's inability to grasp the overly serious nature of the third type, as if their innate life experience were the only "God-given" one—but they can quickly escalate into more serious conflicts, and sometimes into world-shaking events that have terrible consequences.

None of us holds *the* key to fulfillment and meaning. But each one of us has *a* key. Indeed, as individuals and as humanity, we hold seven keys. If we can learn to approach all seven chakra types with a degree of humility, we can also develop the capacity to listen to one another authentically and to experience ourselves as open systems capable of tolerance and change. When we realize that each type has a certain gift that we cannot give ourselves, we open the doors to constructive change and a more harmonious existence. That is the beauty of this system. It teaches us that a healthy society requires all types to influence and support each other.

A New Perspective

To me, what distinguishes this personality system from others is that, aside from being a beneficial self-help tool, it also makes a useful statement about our human society and culture. Above all, this is a *social system* that bears social implications.

Once you study and embrace the chakra types as the basis of personality, you can never look at the world in the same way. It quickly becomes a sort of "built-in" worldview that colors both your internal dialogue—the way you understand yourself—and your interactions with other people. Moreover, it can deeply affect the way you understand social, cultural, and even political phenomena. You may find yourself watching a movie and thinking, "This is such a great fourth-chakra drama." Or you may listen to a musical piece and say, "What a beautiful second-type transmission." Or hear some speaker and sigh, "A natural-born fifth type!"

You begin to identify groups, sectors, and nations as "chakra types" that are all necessary in a complete culture. The world seen through the eyes of the personality types reveals each group's, each nation's, and each religion's gifts to humanity as a whole. These are, of course, gross generalizations; clearly, any nation or cultural movement contains many chakra-type expressions. But remember that this is true for you as well. Your personality cannot be rigidly categorized into only one expression either, and yet each personality has a core activity and inclination. And collective structures and mind-sets have them as well.

We can easily observe cultural phenomena of the second type in eras like the cultural revolution of the sixties, which included a sexual revolution, the discovery of psychedelic substances, music as a form of salvation, and the concept of individual freedom. We can see them in books like *Alice's Adventures in Wonderland*. Berlin is an example of a second-type city—artistic, sexually experimental, highly individualistic, very open, cosmopolitan and pluralistic, relaxed and also quite lazy, and relatively poor because it is generally less driven to rush forward toward progress. Many of its citizens are constantly in search of new experiences and are unable to commit. They are more into the "now" of things, focused on allowing space for self-exploration.

On the other hand, we can easily recognize cultural phenomena of the third type in the era of the samurai in Japanese culture, in Richard Wagner's operas, and in the ancient Greek philosophy of self-mastery. Our wisest path is to focus on the gifts and advantages of each of these cultural phenomena and be inspired by them. Focusing instead on the inevitable excesses they may demonstrate is missing the whole point.

A healthy society will see cultural and individual expressions for what they are—for what they can give and are meant to give—and not for what they are not—what they cannot give. Thinkers think for us all, and thus help stimulate our own minds, while Builders like road workers make it possible for us to drive safely. While some claim that the second type seems somewhat "nonessential," what would our world look like without feelings, sensuality, and poetry? Without humor, laughter, enjoyment, relaxation in the "now," and the creativity of the second type, we would find ourselves in a lifeless march toward a colorless future. The jumpy second type can save us from the overly serious nature of all the other six types. When we come upon a second-chakra type, it is like stumbling upon a beautiful butterfly while in the midst of depression. Our society needs Artists in order to hear, from time to time, that life as it is has its own purpose.

Precisely because none of us can give equal energy and attention to all elements of life, we have to depend on other types to complement and complete our efforts. Do we really want all others to be like us? Imagine the world as eight billion yous—wouldn't that be a nightmare? For our own good, deep down, we need and should want others to be themselves—which means different and contradictory. Admitting this is a first step toward world peace.

There are two types of acceptance to consider. The first is nondiscriminating and impersonal—you accept simply because everyone is equal in the eyes of God, or from a humanistic perspective. The way I see it, however, this is too easy. Our real challenge still awaits us. We must learn to accept people not because they are *not* different, but precisely because they *are*. As long as we are not able to do so, we will suffer from a strange duality in which people generally agree on the reality of human equality, yet, in actual relationships, cannot accept anyone different from themselves.

When we only see people through a lens of equality, this keeps us in an immature state in which we try to overlook differences. Ironically, sometimes the unifying view that claims to believe in equality only makes our intolerance worse. We may still be subtly annoyed because we want to change all others into ourselves. We become truly mature when we love others *because* they are themselves—when we actually enjoy the fact that they perceive and experience differently from the way we do. Our drive to oneness is simply not enough, as long as we cannot see the other as "other."

Both types of acceptance—the recognition of our oneness and the recognition of our differences—are required for perfect relationships, as well as for a healthy society. We reach our highest fulfillment when we realize that the differences we perceive are also a part of the oneness we pursue. The fact that we have elephants, giraffes, lizards, and hippos in the world is not only a wonderful expression of our one indivisible reality, but also an acknowledgment that "God" is even more "God" *because* there are elephants, lizards, and hippos in the world. Diversity does not diminish our oneness; it makes it richer. So we must not minimize it or fear it.

Are the different religions or the different nations of the world meant to merge or disappear simply so that we can finally experience oneness? The chakra types' answer is clearly "No." We don't need to blur national characteristics or blend separate religions just because they appear to create distinctions. Transcending religion and nationality does not mean dissolving them, but rather including them within oneness.

The seven essences embodied by the seven chakra types can serve as a key to the unity of all spiritual systems and religions. While we may think that they contradict each other—of course, all the while vaguely agreeing that they somehow speak of the same "God"—we really need to begin considering them as reflections of different divine aspects. In other words, if we gathered all the different religions and spiritual streams of our world and thoroughly mixed them together, we would get the one true religion.

Evolving Society

When I speak of the seven types in world population, I am often asked if, as humanity evolves, there will be a change in the ratio between the different types. In other words, if there will be fewer Builders and more Thinkers and Yogis in the future. Honestly, I suspect that behind this seemingly intellectual interest lurks an underlying belief that Builders are just a less evolved form of humans. In reality, the ratio between the types makes not relative but inherent sense. It reflects a natural structure in which many are inclined to build and construct our world, since it is, after all, a material world that demands the creation of solid and carefully cultivated realities. Can we really imagine a world crowded with dreamy idea-makers and relaxed and indifferent meditators?

We need only one Socrates to formulate ethics and teach us right thinking, and it is perfectly fine that millions of people follow in his footsteps. We surely don't need everyone to operate in the realm of pure ideas. From my own observation of cultural development and division, I feel that it is the general tendency of culture to arrange itself and take form in response to the actual needs of the world. From a purely practical perspective, for the world to "happen," we require more Builders, Achievers, Speakers, and Caretakers than we do Artists, Thinkers, and Yogis.

On the other hand, our world as it is suffers from the excesses of some of the types. We know very well by now that when each type acts egotistically, it becomes destructive. Yet certain types— the third and fifth types in particular—are more dangerous than others when allowed to remain imbalanced. But although Speakers and Achievers are capable of bringing great destruction into the world, they also hold the key to actualizing an ideal society. More than all others, they are able to give humanity the best future it can have when they act responsibly.

Our system of education has been manipulated—in this case, by Speakers and Achievers—to reinforce the divisions in society. In a cultural form of survival of the fittest, everything is graded and everyone is ranked, with the victorious being hailed and the weak being humiliated. In an ideal society, on the other hand, each type would enjoy full recognition of their nature and, accordingly, an opportunity to cultivate their own being. At the same time, they would be trained to embrace all other qualities as balancing elements. Each type would be allowed to develop both individually and holistically. All seven types would be encouraged, with second types enriching the children with the spirit of laughter and poetry, recognizing the beauty of life in the moment, and promoting the art of enjoyment, while seventh types would teach them meditation, silence, and consciousness.

A truly "enlightened" society will skillfully integrate all seven types without a hierarchy of values, combining all their gifts toward one goal—the goal of peace. It would encourage all types to collaborate in a way that goes beyond self-interest and mere individual expression. Currently, each type just pushes forward its own values, with the third and fifth types monitoring the entire process. The result is that each type contributes only indirectly to society. Because everyone strives to express themselves, our culture is somehow the sum total of all individual impulses. A more conscious society would demonstrate a reality in which all individuals are important—for the sake of the whole.

The chakras are great collaborators. All seven of them "know" very well that to create the complex and marvelous symphony of human life, they need each other. Without the ideal teamwork that helps them synchronize, however, our chakra system would be more like an orchestra in which one violinist plays without caring about the overall composition. To produce a perfect melody in our lives, we must have all seven chakras balanced and aligned. Each of them holds the power to cool down or enhance, to elevate or push forward all the others; each of them may be the solution to another chakra's problems and imbalances. Like seven best friends who support one another along a shared journey, the chakras depend heavily on each other to form one flow of health, peace, intelligence, and consciousness.

This is the genius of the chakras. As different centers of perception and experience that combine into one human being, they can demonstrate a sort of utopian community. For this reason, when we establish an optimal communion within our own chakra system, we can attain inner peace. This inner peace can then serve as a standard for a larger, more external peace—a harmony between our own chakra type and other types, and as a profound mutual understanding, acceptance, and collaboration in the world at large.

BIBLIOGRAPHY

General Sources

Cousens, Gabriel. *Spiritual Nutrition*. Berkley: North Atlantic
    Books, 2005.
Love, Presley. Universe of Symbolism. *http://www.universeofsymbolism*
    .com/chakra-animals.html, accessed October 11, 2017.
Mercier, Patricia. *The Chakra Bible*. New York: Sterling, 2007.

CHAPTER 1: First Chakra—The Builders

Creel, H. G. *Confucius: The Man and the Myth*. Whitefish, MT:
    Kessinger Publishing, 2008.
Lewis, Rick. "Kant 200 Years On," *Philosophy Now*, 49: 2005.
https://www.brainyquote.com/authors/confucius.

CHAPTER 2: Second Chakra—The Artists

Norton, Charlie. "The Man Who Fell to Earth," *Daily Mail Online*,
    June 2012.
https://www.biography.com/people/jim-morrison-9415576.
https://www.brainyquote.com/authors/jim_morrison.

CHAPTER 3: Third Chakra—The Achievers

Nietzsche, Friedrich. *The Will to Power*. Ed., Walter Kaufmann;
    trans., R. J. Hollingdale. New York: Vintage Books, 2011.

Plutarch. *The Life of Alexander the Great.* Ed., Arthur Hugh
    Clough; trans., John Dryden. New York: Modern Library,
    2004.
https://www.brainyquote.com/authors/alexander_the_great.

CHAPTER 4: Fourth Chakra—The Caretakers

Plato. *Phaedrus.* Trans., Christopher Rowe. New York: Penguin
    Classics, 2005.
https://www.biography.com/people/mother-teresa-9504160.
https://www.goodreads.com/author/quotes/838305.Mother_Teresa.

CHAPTER 5: Fifth Chakra—The Speakers

Dawkins, Richard. *The Selfish Gene.* United Kingdom: Oxford
    University Press, 1989.
King Jr., Martin Luther. *The Autobiography of Martin Luther King,
    Jr.* Ed., Clayborne Carson. New York: Warner Books, 1998.
http://www.biographyonline.net/spiritual/osho.html.
https://www.brainyquote.com/authors/martin_luther_king_jr.

CHAPTER 6: Sixth Chakra—The Thinkers

Keller, Evelyn Fox. *A Feeling for the Organism: The Life and Work of
    Barbara McClintock.* New York: Henry Holt and Company,
    1984.

CHAPTER 7: Seventh Chakra—The Yogis

https://en.wikipedia.org/wiki/Anandamayi_Ma.
https://www.goodreads.com/author/quotes/936645.Anandamayi_Ma.

ABOUT THE AUTHOR

Shai Tubali is an international author, thinker, and speaker in the fields of self-development, popular psychology, philosophy, yoga, and spirituality. He is the head of the Human Greatness Center, a holistic health center in Berlin, where he leads seminars on spiritual transformation and psychological development. Shai has led workshops and retreats in Israel, Germany, and India. He is also the developer of transformative methods 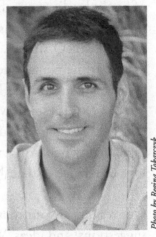 that mix meditation, therapy, and self-empowerment and that are applied by psychologists and therapists throughout Europe. Visit him at *shaitubali.com.*

Photo by Regina Tokarczyk